Polymers for Pharmaceutical Application

药用高分子材料

（中文导读版）

刘 黎　郭圣荣　主编

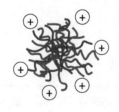
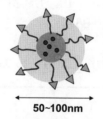

50~100nm

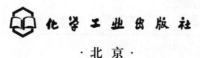

化学工业出版社

·北京·

药用高分子材料是药物制剂不可缺少的物质基础，系统学习了解药用高分子材料相关知识，是现代药学科技工作者，尤其是药剂学专业学生的迫切需要。

本书是编者总结十余年的教学经验，参考大量英文原版文献和书籍并选取适合教学大纲要求的内容编写而成，主要内容以英文编写，并对关键知识点配以中文导读，便于学生阅读和理解。全书共分 6 章，内容包括：药用辅料概述；高分子材料概述；常用天然高分子辅料和合成高分子辅料的结构、性质及其在药剂学中的应用；新型生物可降解的合成药用高分子材料；最后介绍了新型药物输送体系中的药用水凝胶材料、纳米制剂与自组装高分子、高分子-药物轭合物和高分子基因载体。

本书可作为药学专业本科生教材和药剂学专业研究生参考教材，也可供药学、医学和高分子材料学等方面的科技工作者参考。

图书在版编目 (CIP) 数据

Polymers for Pharmaceutical Application——药用高分子材料（中文导读版）/刘黎，郭圣荣主编. —北京：化学工业出版社，2015.1

ISBN 978-7-122-21813-1

Ⅰ. ①P…　Ⅱ. ①刘…　②郭…　Ⅲ. ①药物学-高分子材料-教材-英、汉　Ⅳ. ①R9②TB324

中国版本图书馆 CIP 数据核字（2014）第 210000 号

责任编辑：翁靖一　　　　　　　　　　　　　装帧设计：韩　飞
责任校对：宋　玮

出版发行：化学工业出版社（北京市东城区青年湖南街 13 号　邮政编码 100011）
印　　刷：北京永鑫印刷有限责任公司
装　　订：三河市宇新装订厂
710mm×1000mm　1/16　印张 11　字数 209 千字　　2015 年 1 月北京第 1 版第 1 次印刷

购书咨询：010-64518888（传真：010-64519686）　　售后服务：010-64518899
网　　址：http://www.cip.com.cn
凡购买本书，如有缺损质量问题，本社销售中心负责调换。

定　　价：49.00 元

前 言
Foreword

近年来，许多高校开展了采用汉语和英语的双语教学实践，这对办学国际化和国际化办学很重要，也是培养具有国际竞争力的高素质人才的需要。

随着药用新材料的发展对药物输送系统和技术的不断促进，国际上对药用高分子材料的研究也越来越受到人们的关注。系统学习了解药用高分子材料相关知识，是现代药学科技工作者、尤其是药剂学专业学生的迫切需要。但目前，还没有一本适合药用高分子材料课程的双语教材。国际上，这一领域符合教学要求的英文原版书籍也很匮乏，国外第一本作为教材使用的《Polymers in Drug Delivery》于 2006 年才由 CRC 出版社出版。若在教学中直接采用英文原版教材，价格不菲，学生对于大量专业名词术语的理解也有困难。本教材《Polymers for Pharmaceutical Application——药用高分子材料（中文导读版）》就是为了适应双语教学的新形势和课程要求而编写的。希望本书的出版可以填补药用高分子材料双语教学教材的空白，有助于双语教学过程的规范。学生阅读英文版内容并对照关键知识点的中文导读，可以接触和掌握大量专业词汇，对药学专业本科生的专业英文水平提高一定有所裨益。

编者先后在复旦大学和上海交通大学药学院讲授药用高分子材料课程 10 余年。本教材以编者多年的教学经验为基础，参考大量英文原版文献和书籍，根据我国教学大纲的要求编写而成。全书共分 6 章，主要内容如下：第 1 章为药用辅料概述；第 2 章为高分子材料概述；第 3 章、第 4 章分别介绍选材于《Handbook of Pharmaceutical Excipients》（6th Edition, edited by Raymond C Rowe, Paul J Sheskey and Paul J Weller）中的天然高分子辅料和合成高分子辅料，包括它们的结构、性质及其在药剂学中的应用；第 5 章介绍现代药物输送系统研发中涉及的合成类生物可降解高分子材料；第 6 章介绍功能高分子材料在新型药物输送体系中应用进展的几个热点方向，包括：药用水凝胶材料、纳米制剂与自组装高分子、高分子-药物轭合物、高分子基因载体。每章/节的重点内容均有中文导读，便于学生阅读和理解。

在本书编写过程中，上海交通大学药学院药物控释技术与医药用高分子课题组的沈园园老师，研究生蒋金均、吴可沁、李敏、汪芸，参与了资料收集和整理等工作。英文部分内容得到了上海交通大学外国语学院刘兴华老师的帮助和润色。在此一并表示衷心感谢。

本书可作为药学专业本科生教材和药剂学专业研究生参考教材，也可供药学、医学和高分子材料学等方面的科技工作者参考。

由于药用高分子材料是一个涉及化学、材料、生物、药学和医学的交叉领域，资料的收集整理未必全面，若有疏漏和不完善之处，衷心希望广大读者批评指正。

编者
2014 年 6 月

Chapter 1. Introduction to Pharmaceutical Excipients
药用辅料概述 ·· 1

1.1　Definition of pharmaceutical excipients ······································ 1
1.2　What are excipients doing in medicines? ···································· 2
1.3　Quality and safty of excipients ·· 3
1.4　Relationship between polymers and pharmaceutical excipients ······ 5
1.5　Specific notes for polymers used in drug delivery system ·········· 6
本章中文导读 ··· 7
References ··· 9

Chapter 2. Introduction to Polymers
高分子材料概述 ··· 10

2.1　What are polymers? ·· 10
2.2　Polymer structure and morphology ·· 11
　2.2.1　Molecular weight ·· 11
　2.2.2　Configuration and conformation ·· 12
　2.2.3　Chain structure ·· 14
　2.2.4　Crystalline ·· 15
2.3　Synthesis ··· 17
　2.3.1　Addition polymerization ·· 17
　2.3.2　Condensation polymerization ·· 19
　2.3.3　Cross-linking reaction ··· 19
2.4　Characteristic properties of polymers ······································ 20
　2.4.1　Thermal properties ··· 20
　2.4.2　Mechanical properties ·· 22
　2.4.3　Viscoelastic properties ··· 23

2.5 Characterization techniques ································· 23

  2.5.1 Determination of molecular weight ················ 23

  2.5.2 Determination of structure ·························· 24

  2.5.3 Differential scanning calorimetry ················· 25

2.6 Fabrication and processing ···························· 26

  2.6.1 Injection molding ································ 27

  2.6.2 Extrusion ··· 27

  2.6.3 Spinning ·· 27

本章中文导读 ··· 28

References ·· 32

Chapter 3. Natural Polymers as Pharmaceutical Excipients
天然来源的药用高分子辅料 ················ 33

3.1 Starch and its derivates ····························· 33

  3.1.1 Starch ·· 33

  3.1.2 Pregelatinized starch ····························· 36

  3.1.3 Dextrin ··· 37

  3.1.4 Cyclodextrin ······································ 39

  3.1.5 Sodium carboxymethyl starch ···················· 42

本节中文导读 ··· 44

3.2 Cellulose and its derivates ·························· 46

  3.2.1 Microcrystalline cellulose ························· 46

  3.2.2 Powdered cellulose ································ 47

  3.2.3 Methylcellulose ··································· 48

  3.2.4 Ethylcellulose ···································· 50

  3.2.5 Hydroxyethyl cellulose ···························· 52

  3.2.6 Hydroxypropyl cellulose ·························· 54

  3.2.7 Hydroxypropyl methylcellulose ··················· 56

  3.2.8 Carboxymethylcellulose sodium ·················· 59

  3.2.9 Carboxymethylcellulose calcium ·················· 60

  3.2.10 Cellulose acetate phthalate ······················ 61

本节中文导读 ··· 63

3.3 Other natural polymers in pharmaceutics ············· 66

  3.3.1 Chitin/chitosan ···································· 66

  3.3.2 Alginate and sodium/calcium alginate ·················· 68

  3.3.3 Acacia ··········· 71

  3.3.4 Xanthan gum ········· 72

  3.3.5 Gelatin ·········· 74

  3.3.6 Albumin ········· 76

 本节中文导读·············· 78

 References············ 80

Chapter 4. Synthetic Polymers as Pharmaceutical Excipients
合成的药用高分子敷料 ·················· 81

 4.1 Polymers based on polyvinyl ·············· 81

  4.1.1 Polyvinyl alcohol ··········· 81

  4.1.2 Polymethacrylates ·········· 83

  4.1.3 Polyvinylpyrrolidone (Povidone) ········· 87

  4.1.4 Crospovidone ·········· 89

  4.1.5 Carbomer ·········· 90

 本节中文导读·············· 93

 4.2 Polymers based on polyether·············· 95

  4.2.1 Polyethylene glycol ·········· 95

  4.2.2 Poloxamer ·········· 99

  4.2.3 Polysorbates ·········· 102

 本节中文导读·············· 105

 References············ 106

Chapter 5. Novel Synthetic Biodegradable Polymers as Drug Delivery Carrier
新型可生物降解的合成药用高分子材料 ·················· 107

 5.1 Introduction ··········· 107

 5.2 Polymers based on polyester ·········· 108

  5.2.1 Poly(lactic acid) and poly(lactic-co-glycolic acid) copolymers ·········· 108

  5.2.2 Polycaprolactone ·········· 111

  5.2.3 Poly(β-hydroxybutyrate) ·········· 112

 5.3 Other biodegradable polymers ·········· 113

　　　5.3.1　Poly(orthoesters) ··· 113

　　　5.3.2　Poly(phosphate esters)·· 115

　　　5.3.3　Polyanhydrides ··· 116

　　　5.3.4　Poly(amino acids) ··· 117

　　　5.3.5　Polyphosphazenes ·· 119

　本章中文导读 ·· 121

　References ·· 124

Chapter 6. Advanced Applications of Functional Polymer in Drug Delivery

功能高分子材料在药物输送中的应用进展 ································· 125

　6.1　Hydrogels for pharmaceutical application ························ 125

　　　6.1.1　Introduction ·· 125

　　　6.1.2　Preparation of hydrogels ·· 126

　　　6.1.3　Properties of hydrogels·· 127

　　　6.1.4　Pharmaceutical applications of hydrogels ···················· 129

　本节中文导读 ·· 133

　6.2　Polymer-based nanomedicine and self-assemblying polymers ·········· 134

　　　6.2.1　Introduction to nanomedicine ·································· 134

　　　6.2.2　Micellation of self-assemblying polymers ···················· 134

　　　6.2.3　Biological significance of polymeric micelles ················ 136

　　　6.2.4　Drug release from polymeric micelles ························ 137

　　　6.2.5　Examples of polymeric micelles for drug delivery ············ 138

　本节中文导读 ·· 141

　6.3　Polymer-drug conjugates·· 142

　　　6.3.1　Introduction ·· 142

　　　6.3.2　Design and development of polymer-drug conjugates ·········· 144

　　　6.3.3　Examples for polymer-drug conjugates ······················ 146

　本节中文导读 ·· 152

　6.4　Polymers for gene delivery ·· 153

　　　6.4.1　Introduction to gene delivery ·································· 153

　　　6.4.2　Polymeric vectors ·· 154

　本节中文导读 ·· 161

　References ·· 162

Chapter 1.

Introduction to Pharmaceutical Excipients
药用辅料概述

1.1 Definition of pharmaceutical excipients

Medicines are available in many dosage forms including tablets, capsules, oral liquids, topical creams and gels, transdermal patches, injectable products, implants, inhalers, suppositories and so on. These medicinal products contain not only active drugs but also other ingredients collectively known as excipients. The word *excipient* is derived from the Latin word *excipere*, meaning "to receive, to gather, to take out", which can be simply explained as "other than". Therefore, the United States National Formulary of 1994 states that an excipient is any component other than the active principle added intentionally to the medicinal formulation, or "everything in the formulation except the active drug"[1].

Excipients have been used in drug delivery for centuries. Historically, for example, medicines were often mixed with honey or syrup to mask the flavor so that patients especially children would take them. Other excipients may be added to drugs as diluents to ensure that a medicinal product has the weight, consistency and volume necessary for the correct administration of the active principle to the patient. These usages of excipients are simply to make the product taste and look better and to improve patient compliance. Therefore, prescribers initially overlook excipients as inert substances used as vehicles and diluents for drugs on the assumption that they are inactive.

Ideally, excipients should be inert. However, recent studies in pharmaceutics have suggested otherwise. In reality, these inactive ingredients may facilitate the absorption of a drug into the body, or slow the absorption rate of a drug, or facilitate the breakdown of the drug once it reaches the right area of the body. For example, the drug would dissolve slowly with some excipients in the form of a time release coating. In addition to affecting the biopharmaceutical profile of a drug, excipients also play an important part in the manufacturing process.

Today, pharmaceutical excipients refer to substances that are usually included in a pharmaceutical dosage form not to direct the therapeutic action, but to aid the manufacturing process, to protect, support or enhance stability, or for bioavailability or patient acceptability, to assist in product identification and to enhance the overall safety or function of the product during storage or use. Although technically "inactive" from the therapeutic sense, pharmaceutical excipients are critical and essential components of a modern drug product. It is reported that pharmaceutical excipients represent a market value of about $4 billion accounting for 0.5% of the total pharmaceutical market in 2009[2].

1.2　What are excipients doing in medicines?

Though the active ingredient in a medicine is only part of the arsenal against disease, they are almost never administered alone but in dosage forms that generally include excipients. A drug is desirable to take therapeutic action when it gets to the right place at the right time. That's where drug delivery comes in. Drug delivery is often approached via a drug's chemical formulation, in which pharmaceutical excipients make up the bulk of the total dosage form in many products and exert functions.

Taking the solid form of a tablet as an example, a tablet product must be stable during storage, transport and handling, yet will release its active pharmaceutical ingredient as required once ingested. To achieve the goal, the manufacture of tablets might be a complex process which demands considerable ingenuity involving various excipients, such as diluents or fillers, binders, disintegrants, glidants, lubricants, coloring agents and so on. Table 1-1 presents common excipients used in tablets and their functions.

Dr. Rutesh H. Dave has examined the top 200 prescription tablets and capsules products of 2003, and found out that except coating and coloring agents, the total number of inactive excipients used was ONLY 94 [3]. This finding indicates that an excipient may have more than one use in practice. Moreover, a blend of two or more materials may be necessary as excipients in a product in order to meet the practical requirements. However, it is advisable to reduce the number of excipients needed, so that the risk of interactions among various excipients may be minimized.

In general, excipients are added to formulations in order to improve the bioavailability and the acceptance of the drug on patients. Excipients influence the speed and efficiency of drug absorption, and hence affect drug bioavailability.

Recently, there has been much research on drug delivery systems which aims for greater pharmacological response and minimal side effects. The availability of new drug delivery systems mostly depends on the development of pharmaceutical excipients, which may also allow an extension of patent protection for an active pharmaceutical ingredient.

Table 1-1. Common excipients used in tablets and their functions[2].

Excipient	Function	Examples
Diluents	Provide bulk and enable accurate dosing of potent ingredients	Sugar compounds e.g. lactose, dextrin, glucose, sucrose, sorbitol. Inorganic compounds e.g. silicates, calcium and magnesium salts, sodium or potassium chloride
Binders, compression aids, granulating agents	Bind the tablet ingredients together giving form and mechanical strength	Mainly natural or synthetic polymers e.g. starches and cellulose derivatives
Disintegrants	Aid dispersion of the tablet in the gastrointestinal tract, releasing the active ingredient and increasing the surface area for dissolution	Compounds which swell or dissolve in water e.g. starch, cellulose derivatives and alginates, crospovidone
Glidants	Improve the flow of powders during tablet manufacturing by reducing friction and adhesion between particles. Also used as anti-caking agents.	Colloidal anhydrous silicon and other silica compounds
Lubricants	Similar action to glidants, however, they may slow disintegration and dissolution. The properties of glidants and lubricants differ, although some compounds, such as starch and talc, have both actions.	Stearic acid and its salts (e.g. magnesium stearate)
Tablet coatings and films	Protect tablet from the environment (air, light and moisture), increase the mechanical strength, mask taste and smell, aid swallowing, assist in product identification. Can be used to modify release of the active ingredient. May contain flavours and colorings.	Sugar (sucrose) has now been replaced by film coating using natural or synthetic polymers. Polymers that are insoluble in acid, e.g. cellulose acetate phthalate, are used for enteric coatings to delay release of the active ingredient.
Coloring agents	Improve acceptability to patients, aid identification and prevent counterfeiting. Increase stability of lightsensitive drugs.	Mainly synthetic dyes and natural colours. Compounds that are themselves natural pigments of food may also be used.

1.3 Quality and safty of excipients

A list of excipients included in the medicine is available online in the Consumer Medicine Information leaflet (www.nps.org.au/search_by_medicine_name). Related information can be found under 'Product description' and may be entitled differently as 'Other ingredients' or 'This product also contains⋯'. Ideally, an excipient is pharmacologically inactive, non-toxic, and does not interact with the active ingredients or other excipients. However, in practice adverse effects may be caused by excipients. Toxicity may relate to compounds used as excipients in the final dosage form, or to residues of compounds (such as solvents) used during the manufacturing process.

Components employed as excipients shall not only contain the characteristics required by their technological function as mentioned above, but also meet the suitable safety requirements. However, the importance of evaluating the possible adverse effects of excipients was underestimated in the past, because their inertia and innocuity were taken for granted. The toxicological aspect of these substances has been more deeply studied only when they are also employed in the food industry (as anti-oxidants, sweeteners, coloring agents, etc.). Changes do not come till some excipients were reported to have potential risks. Indeed, the International Toxicological Committees (among which the Joint Expert Committee on Food Additives, a mixed committee of the WHO[●]/FAO) has demanded thorough investigations of excipients in laboratory animals, with the intent of protecting the consumers' safety. Tackling the issue of excipients toxicity thoroughly is not easy for several reasons: the large number of substances on the market and the diversity of their chemical profiles, their sources, their technological functions, and the presence of secondary products and/or contaminants which may otherwise be the true cause for adverse effects[1].

Hence, any material used in pharmaceutical drug product (e.g., excipient, active pharmaceutical ingredient, packaging, etc.) should observe specific standard and shall be manufactured under appropriate Good Manufacturing Practices (GMP) and supplied under Good Distribution Practices (GDP). The exact definition of GMP or GDP will depend on the material in question and legislation where the excipient is supplied or sold.

It is necessary for pharmacists to be familiar with the properties of pharmaceutical excipients. *Handbook of Pharmaceutical Excipients* contains monographs for 340 excipients, with each monograph including a 'Safety' section that introduces adverse reactions reviewed from the literature. This handbook is in the 7th edition updated in 2012[4]. What's more, the Pharmacopoeias (US Pharmacopoeia, British Pharmacopoeia) also contain monographs for many excipients.

International Pharmaceutical Excipients Council (IPEC), an international industry association founded in 1991 by manufacturers and users of excipients, consists of three regional pharmaceutical excipient industry associations covering the United States, Europe, and Japan (which are known respectively as IPEC-Americas, IPEC Europe, and JPEC). IPEC's objective is to contribute to the development and harmonization of international excipient standards, the introduction of useful new excipients to the marketplace and the development of best practice and guidance concerning excipients. *Qualification of Excipients for Use in Pharmaceuticals*, a document published by IPEC in 2008 introduces the three phases of the excipient qualification process. Although excipient qualification does not directly involve regulatory authorities, many conditions need to be satisfied if an excipient is employed in medicine. On the other hand, excipients are diverse and often have uses in areas other than pharmaceutical applications. Thus, this document is especially valuable for suppliers, as many of the issues described on the material are new to them. This document serves as guidelines offering advice and best practice to both excipient suppliers and users. It is not meant

---

[●] Abbr. of World Health Organization.

to be proscriptive, but is intended to be comprehensive covering some essential aspects of the supplier-user relationship.

1.4 Relationship between polymers and pharmaceutical excipients

Many polymers, mainly including cellulose derivatives, poly(ethylene glycol) (PEG), and poly(N-vinyl pyrrolidone) (PVP), have been widely used in drug delivery system as excipients for more than half a century. They are incorporated with bioactive agents in the pharmaceutical industry usually by the techniques such as compression, spray and dip coating, and encapsulation. Recently, some other polymers, such as nano- and micro-particles, nano- and micro-capsules, dendrimers and micelles, have also been tested as potential drug delivery systems, in which the drug is embedded or covalently conjugated in polymer matrices.

From a practical perspective, the use of polymers in pharmaceutical domain falls into two areas: drug polymer and drug carrier polymers for controlled release. Controlled release methods offer an appropriate tool for site-specific and time-controlled delivery of drugs. From a drug delivery perspective, polymer devices can be categorized as diffusion-controlled (monolithic devices), solvent-activated (swelling- or osmotically-controlled devices), chemically controlled (biodegradable), or externally-triggered systems (e.g., pH, temperature) [5]. Mechanisms involved in controlled release require polymers with a variety of physicochemical properties.

At the early beginning, polymers used as pharmaceutical excipients are commonly off-the-shelf materials. Nevertheless, much research effort has been devoted to designing new formulations to achieve a higher desired pharmacological response, where particular attention are paid to the polymeric systems of drug carriers. In fact, the tremendous growth in this field is driven in part by innovations in polymer science and chemical engineering. Particularly, the advanced research in polymer science has provides the clinician with a large number of new materials, new medical device and new formulations[6].

For example, hydrogels and other polymer-based carriers have been developed to provide safe passage for pharmaceuticals through inhospitable physiological regions. Polymers of controlled molecular architecture can be engineered to give a well-defined response to external conditions as a result of a solid understanding of the underlying mechanisms and the nature of behavioral transitions. Polymers incorporated with therapeutics can be bioactive to provide their own therapeutic benefit or can be biodegradable to improve release kinetics and prevent carrier accumulation. Pharmaceutical agents have been conjugated to polymers to modify transport or circulation half-life characteristics as well as to allow for passive and active targeting.

In addition, the latest drug delivery research using polymeric materials has produced recognitive systems that facilitate cytoplasmic delivery of novel therapeutics.

In a word, Modern advances in drug delivery rely on the rational design of polymers tailored for specific cargo and engineered to exert distinct biological functions. Today, drug delivery research has developed into a major interdisciplinary effort involving chemists, biologists, engineers and physicians.

1.5 Specific notes for polymers used in drug delivery system

A crucial feature of polymers used in drug delivery is the mechanism by which they are removed from the body. They may be excreted directly via kidneys (renal clearance) or biodegraded (metabolic clearance) into smaller molecules, which are then excreted. Passage through the renal glomerular membrane is limited to substances with a molecular weight under 50000, although this value varies depending on the chemical structure of the molecule[7]. Molecular weight is especially relevant for substances that are not biodegradable, and macromolecules with a molecular weight lower than the glomerular limit can be safely removed from the body by preventing their accumulation and therefore their potential toxicity.

Another feature of polymers fit in drug delivery is the asepsis. Prior to use, materials must also be sterilized. Agents used to reduce the chances of clinical infection include steam, dry heat, chemicals, and irradiation. Exposing polymers to heat or ionizing radiation may affect the polymer properties, by chain scission or creating cross-links. Chemical agents such as ethylene oxide may also be absorbed by a material and later could be released into the body. Hence, devices sterilized with ethylene oxide require a period of time following sterilization for any residues to be released before use.

◆ **本章中文导读** ◆

一、药用辅料的定义

任何一种药物在供给临床应用时，不可能以原料药形式直接供病人使用，必须制成适合于病人应用的给药形式，如片剂、胶囊剂、注射剂、栓剂、软膏剂等，这种为适应治疗、预防或诊断的需要而制备的不同给药形式通称为药物剂型，简称剂型。药物制剂一般由活性成分的原料和辅料所组成。从药品生产的角度看，药用辅料（pharmaceutical excipients）指除了主要药物活性成分以外一切物料的总称，即为生产药品和调配处方时所用的赋形剂和附加剂。

人类使用药用辅料的历史虽然悠久，但传统意义上的辅料被认为是惰性的，是能将药理活性物质制备成药物制剂的非药理活性成分。近来，随着人们对药物由制剂中释放和被吸收过程的深入了解，已经普遍地认识到：辅料有可能改变药物从制剂中释放的速率和稳定性，从而影响其生物利用度和质量。因此，国际药用辅料协会将辅料定义为：药物制剂中经过合理的安全评价的不包括有效成分或前体的组分。它的作用包括：在药物制剂制备过程中有利于成品的加工；提高药物制剂的稳定性、生物利用度和病人的顺应性；有助于从外观上鉴别药物制剂；改善药物制剂在贮藏或应用时的安全性和有效性。

二、药用辅料的作用

虽然剂型中活性药物是实质性主体部分，决定着作用的整个方向，辅料则保证药物以一定的程序选择性地运送到组织部位，防止药物从制剂释出以前失活，并使药物在体内按一定的速率和时间、在一定的部位释放。以医疗中应用最为广泛的口服固体剂型如片剂、胶囊剂等为例，辅料在制剂中可作为填充材料、黏合性和黏附性材料、崩解性材料、包衣膜材料、保湿性材料、缓控释材料等，同时辅料的加入可改善制剂过程。可见，辅料是制剂生产中必不可少的重要组成部分，在药物制剂的生产中发挥着不可或缺的作用，可以说"没有辅料就没有制剂"。

三、药物辅料的质量和安全性

药物的疗效不仅依赖于其中活性成分的作用，而且与辅料的质量密切相关。从药品安全的角度说，用作药用辅料的材料应该是对人体无毒性、无致敏性、无刺激性、无遗传毒性和无致癌性，对人体组织、血液、免疫等系统不产生不良作用的。实际上完全没有不良作用的材料很难找到，但必须尽量降低材料的不良作用，并使其在人体的忍受范围内。药用辅料的安全性包括：①辅料本身可能的毒性和对人体的不良反应；②材料在合成或加工过程中污染；③辅料和药物或者辅料之间的相互作用导致的不良反应。因此，药用辅料的使用必须经过严格的安全性评价，药用辅料的生产需要进行严格的质量控制。

1991 年成立的国际药用辅料协会 (International Pharmaceutical Excipients Council, IPEC) 致力于药用辅料及其药典标准一体化，管理辅料质量，提出辅料应用的建议，在世界范围内对辅料规范化进行协调，以便于各国之间有关药用辅料的技术交流与合作。在其 2008 版的药用辅料标准中提出了较为详细地对新辅料进行安全性评价的指南。

四、高分子材料与药物辅料的关系

在药剂中发挥重要作用的药用辅料大多是高分子材料。所选用高分子材料的性质及其与药物相互间的作用，决定了药物制剂的性质和质量，控制药物从制剂中的释放行为（释放速率、释放部位、释放的方式如脉冲释放等）。设计和研究新型药物制剂或给药系统取决于新型药用高分子材料的开发。正是许多新的具有特殊性能的高分子材料的出现，诸如口服缓释控释片剂、微球剂、皮下埋植剂以及注射用靶向纳米制剂等现代药物传输系统才得以问世。因此，高分子材料是药物制剂重要的物质基础。

高分子材料作为药用辅料用于药物输送，必须要考虑它如何从体内清除以及无菌化的问题。分子量小于 50000 的材料可以通过肾小球的过滤作用清除体外，或者降解成为小分子被清除[7]。对于在化学性质和物理性质上能够耐受干热或湿热灭菌的高分子材料，采用洁净及无污染的生产条件，在制剂生产过程中加强 GMP 管理以及产品的最终灭菌过程，能满足无菌要求。但对于很多受热不稳定或容易变形的高分子材料，无菌方法的选择直接影响制剂的生物相容性及实际应用。

References

[1] Pifferi G and Restani P. The Safety of Pharmaceutical Excipients. Farmaco, 2003, **58**(8): 541–550.

[2] Haywood A and Glass B D. Pharmaceutical Excipients–Where Do We Begin? Australian Prescriber, 2011, 34(4): 112.

[3] Dave R H. Overview of Pharmaceutical Excipients Used in Tablets and Capsules. Drug Topics, 2008(10).

[4] Rowe R C, Sheskey P J, Cook W G, Fenton M E. Handbook of Pharmaceutical Excipients. 7th Ed. London: Pharmaceutical Press, 2012.

[5] Liechty W B, Kryscio D R, Slaughter B V, Peppas N A. Polymers for Drug Delivery Systems. Annual Review of Chemical and Biomolecular Engineering, 2010, 1: 149.

[6] Dumitriu S. Polymeric Biomaterials, 2nd Ed., Revised and Expanded: New York: Marcel Dekker, Inc., 2001.

[7] Vilar G, Tulla–Puche J, Albericio F. Polymers and Drug Delivery Systems. Current drug delivery, 2012, 9(4): 367–394.

Chapter 2.

Introduction to Polymers
高分子材料概述

2.1 What are polymers?

Polymers are a large class of materials with long-chain molecules that consist of a large number of small repeating units. *Poly-* means "many" and *-mer* means "part" or "segment". Usually, the special name of "monomer" is given to describe those small molecules that can be linked together to form long chains. *Mono* means "one". A typical polymer may contain tens of thousands of monomers. Due to their large size, polymers are classified as macromolecules. "Macro" means "large".

Take polypropylene (PP) for an example: The backbone chain of polypropylene is made up of just two carbon atoms repeated over and over again. One carbon atom has two hydrogen atoms attached to it, and the other carbon atom has one hydrogen atom and one pendant methyl group (CH_3). This is called the *repeat structure* or the *repeat unit*. To the sake of simplicity, the structure of polymer is usually represented as one unit of the repeat structure, as shown in Figure 2-1. The repeat unit is put inside a bracket, and the subscript n just stands for the number of repeat units in the polymer chain.

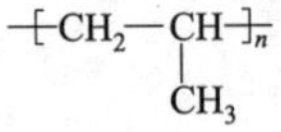

$$-\!\!\left[CH_2-CH\right]_n$$
$$\underset{\displaystyle CH_3}{|}$$

Figure 2-1. Chemical formula of polypropylene schematically.

Polymers may be derived from natural sources, or from synthetic processes. Both natural and synthetic polymers are long-chain molecules that consist of a large number of small repeat units. In synthetic polymers, the chemistry of the repeat units differs from that of the small molecules (monomers) which were used in the original synthesis procedures, resulting from either a loss of unsaturation or the eliminatlion of a small molecule such as water or HCl during polymerization. The exact difference between the monomer and the repeat unit depends on the mode of polymerization, which will be discussed in the following sections.

Historically, people have taken advantage of the versatility of polymers for centuries in the form of oils, tars, resins and gums. However, progress in polymer science was slow until the 1930s, when materials such as vinyl, neoprene, polystyrene and nylon were developed. Polymers are attractive up to now due to the diversity of their properties. Some are rubbery, like a bouncy ball, some are sticky and gooey, and some are hard and tough, like a skateboard. Both natural and synthetic polymers can be produced with a wide range of stiffness, strength, heat resistance, density, and even price. With continued research into the science and applications of polymers, they are playing an ever increasing role in the society.

2.2 Polymer structure and morphology

What makes polymers so fun depends on how their atoms and molecules are connected, which ones are involved in, the degree of polymerization, as well as their physical structure and morphology.

2.2.1 Molecular weight

The fundamental feature of bulk polymers is the degree of polymerization, which can be expressed by molecular weight alternatively. However, unlike a small molecule with a unique molecular weight, a polymer is usually produced with a distribution of molecular weights.

To compare the molecular weights of two different batches of polymers, it is useful to define an average molecular weight. Two useful statistical definitions of molecular weights are the number average and weight average molecular weights. The number average molecular weight (M_n) is the first moment of the molecular weight distribution and is an average over the number of molecules. The weight average molecular weight (M_w) is the second moment of the molecular weight distribution and is an average over the weight of each polymer chain. Equations (2-1) and (2-2) define the two averages:

$$\bar{M}_n = \frac{N_1M_1 + N_2M_2 + N_3M_3 + \cdots + N_nM_n}{N_1 + N_2 + N_3 + \cdots + N_n} = \frac{\Sigma N_iM_i}{\Sigma N_i} \tag{2-1}$$

$$\bar{M}_w = \frac{W_1M_1 + W_2M_2 + W_3M_3 + \cdots + W_nM_n}{W_1 + W_2 + W_3 + \cdots + W_n} = \frac{\Sigma W_iM_i}{\Sigma W_i} \tag{2-2}$$

Where N_i is the number of moles of species i, W_i is the weights of species i and M_i is the molecular weight of species i.

Linear polymers used for biomedical applications generally have M_n in the range of 25000 to 100000 and M_w from 50000 to 300000. In exceptional cases, for example, the M_w of polyethylene used in the hip joint may range up to a million.

Figure 2-2 shows a typical distribution in molecular weight of polymers including the weight and number average molecular weights. The ratio of M_w to M_n is known as the polydispersity index (PI) and is used as a measure of the breadth of the molecular weight distribution. Typical commercial polymers have polydispersity indices of 1.5~5.0, although polymers with polydispersity indices of less than 1.1 can be synthesized with special techniques.

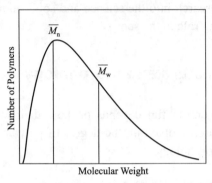

Figure 2-2. Typical curve of molecular weight of polymers.

The molecular weight of a polymer can also be represented by the viscosity average molecular weight (M_v). This form of the molecular weight is found as a function of the viscosity of the polymer in solution, since viscosity determines the flow rate of the solution and the polymer molecular weight influences the viscosity. Using *Mark-Houwink* simulation, the viscosity average molecular weight can be calculated for a specific polymer in a dilute solution of solvent [1].

Mark-Houwink simulation:　$[\eta] = KM^a$

Where K is a constant for the respective material and α is a branching coefficient.

In general, increasing molecular weight of polymers corresponds to increasing physical properties, such as strength, hardness and so on. However, since melt viscosity also increases with molecular weight, process-ability will decrease and an upper limit of useful molecular weights is usually reached. Also, molecular weight may influence the ability of the polymer chains to crystallize and to exhibit secondary interactions such as hydrogen bonding. The crystallinity and secondary interactions can give polymers additional strength.

2.2.2　Configuration and conformation

The structure of a polymer can vary depending on the geometric arrangement of the bonds, an important factor determining the macroscopic properties. Two terms, namely configuration and conformation are used to describe the geometric structure of a polymer, and they are often cause confusions.

Configuration refers to the order that is determined by chemical bonds. The configuration of a polymer cannot be altered unless chemical bonds are broken and reformed. As shown in Figure 2-3, *cis* and *trans* are two types of polymer configurations for polymer chains containing carbon-carbon double bond.

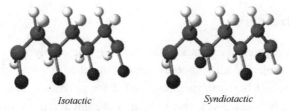

Figure 2-3. Isomers of *cis* and *trans* configurations.

Stereoregularity is another term used to describe the configuration of polymer chains. Three distinct structures can be obtained. *Isotactic* is an arrangement where all substituents are on the same side of the polymer chain. A *syndiotactic* polymer chain is composed of alternating groups and *atactic* is a random combination of the groups. Figure 2-4 shows isostactic and syndiotactic stereoisomers of polypropylene.

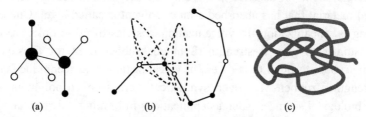

Isotactic   *Syndiotactic*

Figure 2-4. *Stereoisomers* of polymer chain of polypropylene.

Conformation refers to the order that arises from the rotation about single bonds in molecules. If two atoms are joined by a single bond, then rotation about that bond is possible which does not require breaking the bond. The rotation results in an adjustment of the *torsional* angle. If the two atoms have other atoms or groups attached to them as shown in Figure 2-5 (a), then structures which vary in torsional angle are known as *conformations*. It is worth noting that these structures can be changed by physical means (e.g. rotation). Different conformations represent varying distances between the atoms or groups rotating about the bond, which determine the amount and type of interaction between adjacent atoms or groups. Therefore, different conformation may represent different potential energies of the molecule.

Figure 2-5. Rotation of C—C single bonds (a), (b) and random coil of linear polymer (c).

Polymers are usually very long containing many single bonds. Rotations about single bonds [Figure 2-5(b)] will assume the individual polymer molecules many possible conformations. This is the reason that many polymer chains are described as random coil [Figure 2-5 (c)] with flexibility.

A random coil is a polymer conformation describing that the monomer subunits are oriented randomly while still being bonded to adjacent units. It is a statistical distribution of shapes for all the chains in a population of macromolecules. The conformation's name is derived from the idea that, in the absence of specific, stabilizing interactions, a polymer backbone will "sample" all possible conformations randomly. Many linear unbranched homopolymers, in solution or above their melting temperatures, assume (approximate) random coils. Even copolymers with monomers of unequal length will distribute in random coils if the subunits lack any specific interactions.

2.2.3　Chain structure

Most of the polymers we'll talk about here are linear polymers. A linear polymer is made up of one molecule after another, hooked together in a long chain. This chain is called the backbone. It is worth mentioning that for polymers, linear means "straight and not branched", but they don't have to be in a straight and rigid line.

A branched polymer is formed when there are "side chains" (branches) attached to a main chain and thus it has lots of ends. There are many ways for a branched polymer to be arranged, like "star-branching". Star branching can be generated when a polymerization starts with a single monomer and has branches radially outward from this point. Polymers with a high degree of branching are called dendrimers, which tends to be the molecule of an overall spherical shape in three dimensions.

Cross-linking is another specific structure of polymers, in which bonds are formed between neighboring chains in addition to the bonds which hold monomers together in a polymer chain. The so-called "cross-links" can be formed directly between the neighboring chains, or two chains may bond to a third common molecule. These cross-links have an important effect on the properties of polymers. Cross-linked materials neither melt, nor dissolve in solvents, but they can absorb solvents. A piece of cross-linked material that has absorbed a lot of solvent is called a gel. One example of cross-linking is vulcanization. In vulcanization, a series of cross-links are introduced into an elastomer to give it strength. Synthetic rubber used for tires is made by cross-linking rubber through the process of vulcanization. This technique is commonly used to strengthen rubber. Moreover, synthetically cross-linked polymers have many uses in the biological sciences, such as applications in forming polyacrylamide gels for gel electrophoresis. Novel uses for cross-linking can be found in regenerative medicine, where bio-scaffolds are cross-linked to improve their mechanical properties and/or to specifically increase their resistance to dissolution in water based solutions.

What's more, a separate kind of chain structure arises when more than one type of monomer is incorporated into polymer chains. They are known as copolymers. There are three important types of copolymers as shown in Figure 2-6. A random copolymer contains a random arrangement of multiple monomers. A block copolymer consists of blocks of monomers of the same type. Thirdly, a graft copolymer comprises a main chain polymer consisting of one type of monomer with branches made up of other monomers. Normally, random copolymers exhibit properties approximating those of the weighted average of the two types of monomer units, whereas block copolymers tend to phase separate into a monomer-A-rich phase and a monomer-B-rich phase, displaying properties unique to each of the homopolymers.

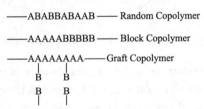

Figure 2-6. Different types of copolymers.

2.2.4 Crystalline

Both molecular shape and the way molecules are arranged on the micro and macroscopic scale in a solid are important factors in determining the properties of polymers. Crystallization, discussed below, is an example of the orientational organizations of molecules into more ordered structures.

Polymers can be either amorphous or semicrystalline. Semi-crystalline means they form mixtures of small crystals and amorphous regions. The crystalline material shows a high degree of order formed by folding and stacking of the polymer chains. The amorphous or glass-like structure shows no long range order, and the chains are tangled. Some polymers are completely amorphous. However, it should be noted that polymers can never be completely crystalline and most are a combination of the tangled and disordered regions surrounding the crystalline areas, as illustrated in Figure 2-7. Therefore, polymers usually melt over a range of temperature instead of at a single melting point. And in most polymers, the combination of crystalline and amorphous structures forms a material with advantageous properties of strength and stiffness.

During the crystallization process, it has been observed that relatively short chains organize themselves into crystalline structures more readily than longer molecules. Hence, the *degree of polymerization* (DP) is an important factor in determining the crystallinity of a polymer. Polymers with a high DP have difficulty in organizing into layers because they tend to become tangled.

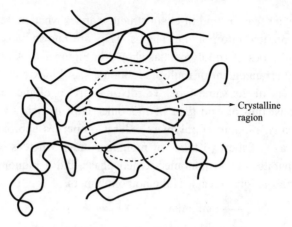

Figure 2-7. Diagram of polymer semicrystalline.

Another factor influencing the polymer morphology is the size and shape of the monomers' substituent groups. If monomers are large and irregular, it is difficult for the polymer chains to arrange themselves in an ordered manner, resulting in a more amorphous solid. Likewise, smaller monomers, and monomers that have a very regular structure (e.g. rod-like) will form more crystalline polymers. The tendency of a polymer to crystallize is enhanced by the small side groups and chain regularity. Atactic polymers usually cannot crystallize, resulting in an amorphous polymer. Isotactic and syndiotactic polymers may crystallize if conditions are favorable.

The cooling rate also influences the amount of crystallinity. Slow cooling provides time for greater amounts of crystallization to occur. On the other hand, fast rates such as rapid quenches, yield highly amorphous materials. Subsequent annealing (heating and holding at an appropriate temperature below the crystalline melting point, followed by slow cooling) will produce a significant increase in crystallinity in most polymers, as well as relieving stresses.

The presence of crystallites in the polymer usually leads to enhanced mechanical properties, unique thermal behavior, and increased fatigue strength. These advantageous properties make semicrystalline polymers desirable materials for biomedical applications. For example, PP is an isotactic crystalline polymer used as sutures. Polyethylene (PE) also possesses a higher level of crystalline structure characterized by folded chain lamellar growth that results in the formation of spherulites. These structures can be visualized in a polarized light microscope.

Low molecular weight polymers (short chains) are generally weaker in strength. Although they are crystalline, only weak Van der Waals forces hold the lattice together. This allows the crystalline layers to slip past one another causing a break in the material. Amorphous polymers with high molecular weight, however, have greater strength because the molecules become tangled between layers. In the case of fibers, stretching to 3 or more times their original length when in a semi-crystalline state produces increased chain alignment, crystallinity and strength.

2.3 Synthesis [2]

Polymer synthesis is a complex procedure and can take place in a variety of ways. Usually, methods of polymer synthesis fall into two categories: addition polymerization (chain reaction) and condensation polymerization (stepwise growth). Ring opening is another type of polymerization and will be discussed in more detail in the section on degradable polymers.

2.3.1 Addition polymerization

Addition polymerization describes the method where unsaturated monomers are added one by one to an active site on the growing chain. There are three significant reactions that take place in addition polymerization: *initiation* (birth), *propagation* (growth), and *termination* (death). The initiators can be free radicals, cations, anions, or stereospecific catalysts. The initiator opens the double bond of the monomer, presenting another "initiation" site on the opposite side of the monomer bond for continuing growth. During the propagation step, rapid chain growth ensues until the reaction is terminated by reaction with another radical, a solvent molecule, another polymer molecule, an initiator, or an added chain transfer agent.

The most common type of addition polymerization is free radical polymerization. As shown in Figure 2-8, free radicals are often created by the division of a molecule (known as an *initiator*) into two fragments along a single bond. In this case, benzoyl peroxide acts as initiator to produce a radical. The radical attacks one monomer, and the electron migrates to another part of the molecule. Then in the propagation stage, this newly formed radical attacks another monomer and the process is repeated. Thus the active center moves down the chain as the polymerization occurs. Here, in free radical polymerization, the entire propagation reaction usually takes place within a fraction of a second. Thousands of monomers are added to the chain within this time. The entire process stops when the termination reaction occurs.

In theory, the propagation reaction could continue until the supply of monomers is exhausted. However, most often the growth of a polymer chain is halted by the termination reaction. Termination typically occurs in two ways: combination and disproportionation, as illustrated in Figure 2-8. Combination occurs when the polymer's growth is stopped by free electrons from two growing chains that join and form a single chain. Disproportionation halts the propagation reaction when a free radical strips a hydrogen atom from an active chain. A carbon-carbon double bond takes the place of the missing hydrogen. Disproportionation can also occur when the radical reacts with an impurity. This is why it is so important that polymerization be carried out under very clean conditions.

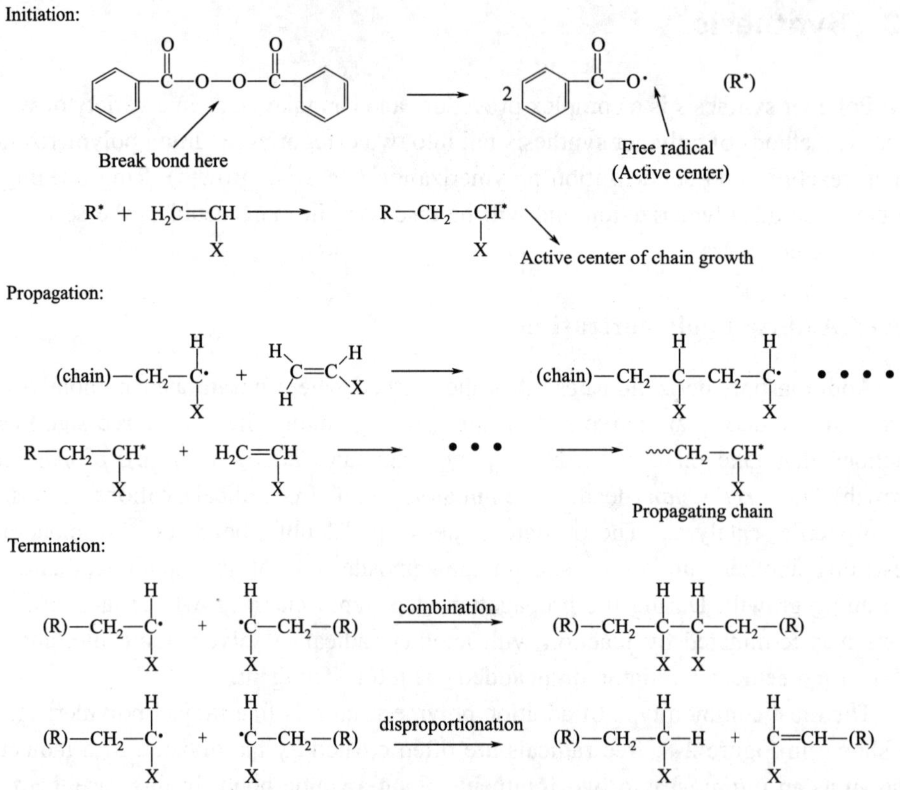

Figure 2-8. Typical process of free radical polymerization.

Molecular weights of polymer chains are difficult to control with precision in free radical polymerization. Added chain transfer agents are used to control the average molecular weights, but molecular weight distributions are usually broad. In addition, chain transfer reactions with other polymer molecules may produce undesirable branched products that affect the ultimate properties of the polymeric material.

Nevertheless, molecular architecture can be controlled very precisely in anionic polymerization, where regular linear chains with PI close to unity can be obtained. It is a type of addition polymerization called "living polymerization", which does not undergo a termination reaction and continues until the monomer supply has been exhausted. And the polymerization will resume, if more monomers are added to the system. Uniform molecular weight (low PI) is characteristic of living polymerization. It also happens in more recent methods of living free radical polymerizations called *atom transfer radical polymerization* (ATRP) and *reversible addition-fragmentation chain transfer* (RAFT). If the supply of monomers and initiator is controlled, the chain length can be manipulated to serve the needs of a specific application.

Polymers produced by addition polymerization can be homopolymers containing only one type of repeat unit, or copolymers with two or more types of repeat units. Depending on the reaction conditions and the reactivity of each monomer type, the copolymers can be random, alternating, graft or block copolymers.

2.3.2   Condensation polymerization

Condensation polymerization is completely analogous to condensation reactions of low-molecular-weight molecules. Two monomers react to form a covalent bond, usually with elimination of a small molecule such as water, hydrochloric acid, methanol or carbon dioxide. The reaction continues until almost all of one reactant is used up. For example, the synthesis of nylon is shown in Figure 2-9 (a), which is a typical condensation polymer used in fiber or fabric form as biomaterials. There are also polymerizations that resemble the stepwise growth of condensation polymers, although no small molecule is eliminated. Polyurethane is a polymer which synthesis bears these characteristics as shown in Figure 2-9 (b).

$$n\,H_2N(CH_2)_6NH_2\ +\ n\,HOOC(CH_2)_4COOH$$

$$\longrightarrow \left[NH(CH_2)_6NH\overset{\overset{O}{\|}}{C}(CH_2)_4\overset{\overset{O}{\|}}{C}\right]_n\ +\ n\,H_2O \qquad\qquad (a)$$

$$n\,HO\!-\!R\!-\!OH\ +\ n\,OCN\!-\!R'\!-\!NCO$$

$$\longrightarrow HO\!\left[R\!-\!OOCNH\!-\!R'\!-\!NHCOO\right]_n\!\!R\!-\!OOCNH\!-\!R'\!-\!NCO \qquad (b)$$

Figure 2-9. Synthesis of nylon-66 (a) and polyurethane (b).

In condensation polymerization, the molecular weight of polymer product can be controlled by the ratio of one reactant to another and by the time of polymerization. The use of bifunctional monomers gives rise to linear polymers, while multifunctional monomers may be used to form covalently cross-linked networks.

2.3.3   Cross–linking reaction

Cross-linking is a chemical process of bonding one polymer chain to another, where a bond that links one polymer chain to another is called a cross-link. Cross-links can be formed by mixing of unpolymerized monomers with specific chemicals called cross-linking reagents. Postpolymerization cross-linking of addition or condensation polymers is also possible. Natural rubber, for example, consists mostly of linear molecules, which can be cross-linked to a loose network with 1%~3% sulfur (vulcanization) or to a hard rubber with 40%~50% sulfur, as shown in Figure 2-10. Properties of the resulting cross-linked polymers depend strongly on the cross-link density.

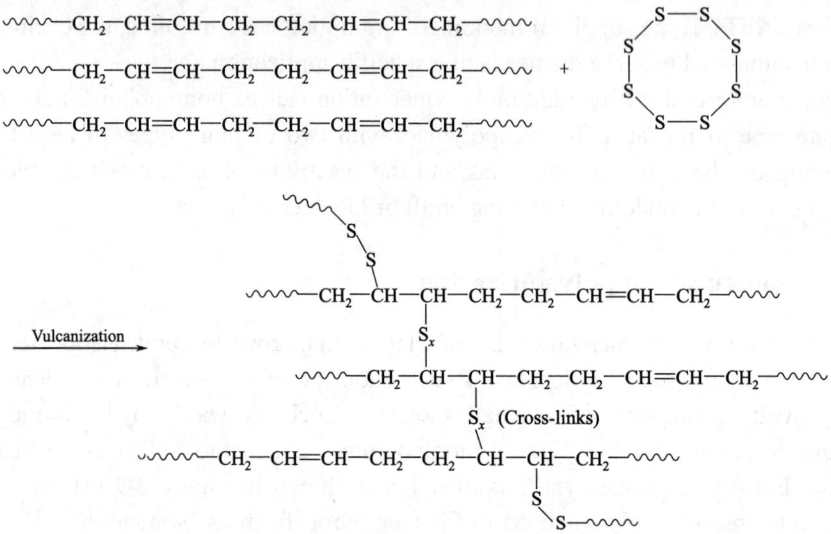

$$\text{\textasciitilde\textasciitilde}-CH_2-CH=CH-CH_2-CH_2-CH=CH-CH_2-\text{\textasciitilde\textasciitilde}$$

$$\text{\textasciitilde\textasciitilde}-CH_2-CH=CH-CH_2-CH_2-CH=CH-CH_2-\text{\textasciitilde\textasciitilde} \quad +$$

$$\text{\textasciitilde\textasciitilde}-CH_2-CH=CH-CH_2-CH_2-CH=CH-CH_2-\text{\textasciitilde\textasciitilde}$$

(S₈ ring structure)

$\xrightarrow{\text{Vulcanization}}$

$$\text{\textasciitilde\textasciitilde}-CH_2-CH-CH-CH_2-CH_2-CH=CH-CH_2-\text{\textasciitilde\textasciitilde}$$
with S_x cross-link to
$$\text{\textasciitilde\textasciitilde}-CH_2-CH-CH-CH_2-CH_2-CH=CH-CH_2-\text{\textasciitilde\textasciitilde}$$
S_x (Cross-links)
$$\text{\textasciitilde\textasciitilde}-CH_2-CH=CH-CH_2-CH_2-CH-CH-CH_2-\text{\textasciitilde\textasciitilde}$$
with S—S—

Figure 2-10. Schematic process of vulcanization.

2.4　Characteristic properties of polymers [3]

2.4.1　Thermal properties

The thermal behaviors of polymers are usually classified by their viscoelastic responses related to temperature. The modulus versus temperature curves, shown in Figure 2-11, illustrate typical behaviors of linear amorphous, cross-linked and semi-crystalline polymers.

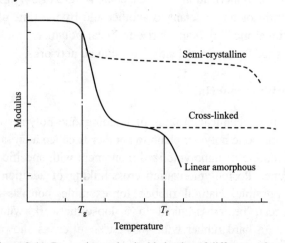

Figure 2-11. Dynamic mechanical behavior of different polymers.

For linear amorphous polymers, their moduli are relatively high at glassy state. Increasing temperature induces the onset of the glass transition region where the modulus drops by three orders of magnitude, and the polymer is transformed from a stiff glass to a leathery material. Here arises an important concept of the glass transition temperature (T_g), which is usually presented in a 5~10℃ temperature span depending on heating rate. The relatively constant modulus region above T_g is the rubbery plateau region where thermal energy is enough for long-range segment of polymer to move randomly (Brownian motion) but is insufficient to overcome entanglement interactions that inhibit flow. Finally, at high enough temperatures, the polymer begins to flow, and a sharp decrease in modulus is seen over a narrow temperature range. The so-called viscous flow temperature (T_f) is the temperature at which the polymer begins to flow. Therefore, temperatures above T_f are the region where polymers are processed into various shapes depending on their end usage.

Semicrystalline polymers exhibit the same general features in modulus versus temperature curves as amorphous polymers. However, they possess a higher plateau modulus owing to the reinforcing effect of the crystallites. Semicrystalline polymers will also exhibit a melting temperature (T_m) owing to melting of the crystalline phase. All polymers have a T_g, but only polymers with regular chain architecture can pack well, crystallize, and exhibit a T_m. The T_g is always below the T_m.

Unlike linear polymers, chemically cross-linked polymers do not display flow behavior. The cross-links inhibit flow at all temperatures below the degradation temperature. Thus, chemically cross-linked polymers cannot be melt processed. These materials are usually processed as reactive liquids or high-molecular-weight amorphous gums that are cross-linked during molding to give the desired product. Some cross-linked polymers are formed as networks during polymerization, and then must be machined into useful shapes. The soft contact lens, composed of poly (hydroxyethyl methacrylate) (PHEMA), is an example of this type of network polymer, which is shaped in the dry state and used when swollen with water.

In general, the thermal transitions in polymers, including T_g, T_f and so on, can be measured by differential scanning calorimetry (DSC), which will be discussed in the section on characterization techniques. Especially, in the study of polymers and their applications, it is important to understand the concept of the glass transition temperature (T_g). T_g is defined as the temperature at which the mechanical properties of a plastic radically changed due to the internal movement of the polymer chains. As the temperature of a polymer drops below T_g, it tends to be hard and glassy. As the temperature rises above the T_g, the polymer becomes more rubber-like. Thus, knowledge of T_g is essential in the selection of materials for various applications. For example, polyvinyl chloride (PVC) has a T_g of 83℃, and will be a brittle solid at room temperature. It makes PVC good, for example, for cold water pipes, but unsuitable for hot water. Adding a small amount of *plasticizer* to PVC can lower the T_g to −40℃. This addition renders the PVC a soft and flexible material at room temperature, ideal for applications as garden hoses. Otherwise, a PVC hose would become stiff and brittle in winter. Overall, the relation of the T_g to the ambient temperature is what determines the choice of a given material in a particular application.

2.4.2 Mechanical properties

The mechanical properties of polymers can be characterized by their deformation behavior. Figure 2-12 shows the stress-strain response of polymers in tensile testing, where a dog-bone-shaped polymer sample is subjected to a constant elongation or strain rate, and the force required to maintain the constant elongation rate is monitored. Glasssy and semicrystalline polymers have higher moduli and lower extensibilities. Amorphous, rubbery polymers are soft and reversibly extensible. They tend to exhibit a lower modulus, and extensibilities of several hundred percent, since the motion freedom of the polymer chain is retained at a local level while large-scale movement or flow is prevented by the chain entanglements and a network structure resulting from chemical cross-linking. Meanwhile, rubbery materials may also exhibit an increase of stress prior to breakage as a result of strain-induced crystallization assisted by molecular orientation in the direction of stress.

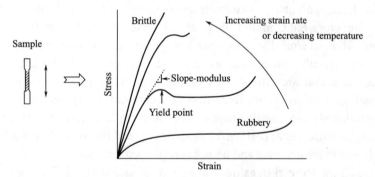

Figure 2-12. The stress-strain response of polymers in tensile testing.

The ultimate strength of polymers is the stress at or near failure. For most materials, failure is catastrophic (complete breakage). However, for some semicrystalline materials, the failure point may be defined by the stress point where large inelastic deformation starts (yielding). The toughness of a polymer is related to the energy absorbed at failure and is proportional to the area under the stress-strain curve.

It is noted that the mechanical property of polymers is strongly related to their temperatures. To know the mechanical properties of polymers are important in selecting particular polymers for biomedical applications.

2.4.3 Viscoelastic properties

The response of materials to the application of a force can be indicated by two main types of behavior: *elastic* and *plastic*. Elastic materials will return to their original shape once the force is removed. Plastic materials will not regain their shape, in which flow is occurring much like a highly viscous liquid. Most polymers demonstrate a combination of elastic and plastic behavior, under mechanical stress, that is so-called viscoelastic behavior which is intermediate between liquids and solids in character. Polymers usually show plastic behavior after the elastic limit has been exceeded.

The viscoelastic properties of polymers depend on many variables, such as temperature, pressure and time. A striking example of the rate dependence of these viscoelastic properties is furnished by Silly Putty. As shown in Figure 2-13, Silly Putty in (a) stretches well by slowly pulling, while it is shattered under quick hitting with a hammer. These images are representative of the behavior of a material above and below its glass transition temperature. The speed of the hammer raised the rate of the application of the force and in turn raised the T_g. This caused the Silly Putty to react as if it were below its T_g and to shatter. Even though both reactions took place at the same ambient temperature, one reaction appeared to be above the effective T_g and the other appeared to be below.

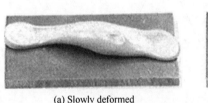

(a) Slowly deformed   (b) Rapidly deformed

Figure 2-13. Images of Silly Putty.

A further complication arises in dealing with general polymers from their semi-crystalline morphology in which amorphous regions and crystalline regions are intermingled. This gives rise to a mixed behavior depending on the percent crystallinity and on their temperature relative to T_g of the amorphous regions.

2.5 Characterization techniques

2.5.1 Determination of molecular weight

Molecular weights of polymers can be measured by gel permeation chromatography (GPC). GPC is a type of size exclusion chromatography, which involves passage of a dilute polymer solution over a column of porous beads. As shown in Figure 2-14, high-molecular-weight polymers are excluded from the beads and elute first, whereas lower molecular-weight molecules pass through the pores of the bead, increasing their elution time. By monitoring the effluent of the column as a function of time using a refractive index or light scattering detector, the amount of polymer eluted during each time interval can be determined. Then the molecular weight of polymer can be determined by comparison of the elution time of the samples with those of monodisperse samples of known molecular weight. Figure 2-15 shows a typical GPC trace.

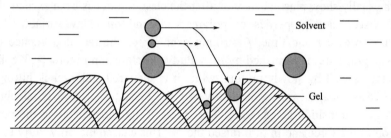

Figure 2-14. Schematic mechanism of GPC.

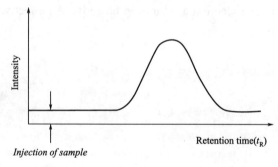

Figure 2-15. A typical GPC curve of polymer.

There are a number of other techniques which can be used to determine the molecular weights of polymers. Those methods such as end-group analysis, vapor pressure osmometry and so on, can be used to measure M_n. Light-scattering techniques are recently emerging to determine M_w. In dilute solution, the scattering of light is directly proportional to the number of molecules. The intensity of the scattered light depends on the polarizability and the polarizability depends on the molecular weight. Therefore, light scattering experiments can be used to measure weight average molecular weight.

2.5.2　Determination of structure

Infrared (IR) spectroscopy and nuclear magnetic resonance (NMR) is often used to characterize the chemical structure of polymers. The analysis is similar as that used in organic chemistry. NMR may also be used in a number of more specialized applications relating to intermolecular interactions of polymers.

Wide-angle X-ray scattering (WAXS) technique is useful for probing the local structure of a semicrystalline polymeric solid. Under appropriate conditions, crystalline materials diffract X-rays, giving rise to spots or rings. According to Bragg's law, these can be interpreted as interplanar spacings. The interplanar spacings can be used without further manipulation or the data can be fit to a model such as a disordered helix or an extended chain. The crystalline chain conformation and atomic placements can then be accurately inferred.

Small-angle X-ray scattering (SAXS) is used in determining the structure of many multiphase materials. This technique requires an electron density difference to be present between two components in the solid and has been widely applied to to study the morphology of copolymers. It can probe features of 10~1000Å in size, and with appropriate modeling of the data, SAXS can give detailed structural information unavailable with other techniques.

2.5.3 Differential scanning calorimetry

Differential scanning calorimetry (DSC) is a method for probing thermal transitions of polymers. As illustrated in Figure 2-16, a sample cell and a reference cell are supplied energy at varying rates so that the temperatures of the two cells remain equal. The thermal properties of a sample are compared against a standard reference material which has no transition in the temperature range of interest, such as powdered alumina. When the temperature is increased, typically at a rate of 10~20°C/min over the range of interest, the energy input required to maintain equality of temperature in the two cells is recorded. Plots of energy supplied versus average temperature allow determination of T_g, crystallization temperature (T_c), and T_m.

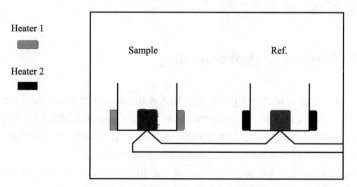

Figure 2-16. Schematic illustration of DSC.

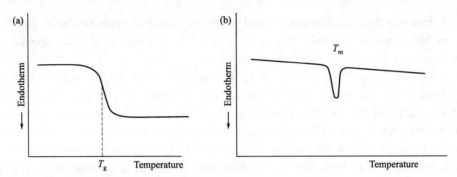

Figure 2-17. The typical DSC curves showing the thermal transitions of polymers.

As illustrated in Figure 2-17(a), a glassy polymer which does not crystallize is being slowly heated from below T_g. T_g is taken as the temperature at which one half the change in heat capacity has occurred. Here, the drop marked T_g at its midpoint represents the increase in energy supplied to the sample to maintain it at the same temperature as the reference material. The sample has the relatively increasing heat capacity as its temperature is raised through T_g. The addition of heat energy corresponds to this endothermal direction.

The T_m is easily identified, as shown in Figure 2-17(b). A melting process is illustrated for the case of a highly crystalline polymer which is slowly heated through its melting temperature. Again, as the melting temperature is reached, an endothermal peak appears because heat must be preferentially added to the sample to continue this essentially constant temperature process. The peak breadth is primarily related to the size and degree of perfection of the polymer crystals. The areas under the peak can be quantitatively related to enthalpic change.

Note that if the process is reversed so that the sample is being cooled from the melt, the plot would be inverted. In that case, as both are being cooled by ambient conditions, even less heat would need to be supplied to the sample than to the reference material, in order that crystals can form. This corresponds to an exothermal process, where T_c can be identified.

2.6 Fabrication and processing

Once a polymer with the right properties is produced, it must be manipulated into some useful shape or object. Various methods are used in industry to do this. Polymers can be fabricated into sheets, films, rods, tubes, and fibers, as coatings on another substrate, and into more complex geometries and foams.

The processing can be achieved using the high-molecular-weight polymer at the start. It is worth noting that the properties of crystalline polymers are sensitive to processing history. Crystalline polymers tend to be tough and ductile plastics. When heated above their flow point, they can be melt processed and will crystallize and become rigid again upon cooling.

Alternatively, polymer products can be fabricated into end-use shapes starting from the monomers or low-molecular-weight prepolymers. In such processes, the final polymerization step is carried out once the precursors are in a casting or molding device, yielding a solid and shaped end product.

2.6.1　Injection molding

One of the most widely used forms of plastic processing is injection molding. Basically, a plastic is heated above its glass transition temperature (enough so that it will flow) and then is forced under high pressure to fill the contents of a mold. The molten plastic is usually "squeezed" into the mold by a ram or a reciprocating screw. The plastic is allowed to cool and is then removed from the mold in its final form. The advantage of injection molding is speed, in which the process can be performed many times each second.

2.6.2　Extrusion

Extrusion is also a method widely used to process plastics, similar to injection molding. In extrusion process, the plastic is heated and forced through a die rather than into a mold. However, the disadvantage of extrusion is that the objects made must have the same cross-sectional shape. Plastic tubing and hose are produced in this manner.

2.6.3　Spinning

Spinning is the process used to produce fibers. There are three main types of spinning: melt, dry and wet. Melt spinning is used for polymers that can be melted easily. Dry spinning involves dissolving the polymer into a solution that can be evaporated. Wet spinning is used when the solvent cannot be evaporated and must be removed by chemical means. All types of spinning use the same principle, so it is convenient to just describe one in details. In melt spinning, a mass of polymer is heated until it will flow. The molten polymer is pumped to the face of a metal disk containing many small holes, called the spinneret. Tiny streams of polymer that emerge from these holes (called filaments) are wound together as they solidify, forming a long fiber. Speeds of up to 750 m/min can be employed in spinning.

Following the spinning process, as noted in the section on polymer crystalline, fibers are stretched substantially——from 3 to 8 or more times their original length to produce increased chain alignment and enhanced crystallinity in order to yield improved strength.

◆ **本章中文导读** ◆

一、高分子的概念

高分子材料在人们的现代生活中随处可见，如品种繁多的塑料制品、橡胶轮胎、衣服织物、隐形眼镜……，甚至人自身的肌体，也包含大量的蛋白质、核酸等生物高分子。高分子（polymer）是高分子量化合物的简称，就是那些分子量特别大的化合物。高分子一般由几千、几万甚至几十万个原子组成，分子量为 10^4～10^6。高分子的"高"就是指它的分子量高。通常将生成高分子的那些小分子原料称为单体（monomer）。一个大分子往往由许多简单的结构单元通过共价键重复键接而成，大分子链上这些化学组成和结构均可重复的最小单位，简称重复单元。许多重复单元连接成线型大分子，类似一条链子，重复单元的数目叫聚合度（degree of polymerization，简称 DP），重复单元俗称作链节。

二、高分子的结构

高分子的结构非常复杂，包括高分子链的近程结构，如结构单元的化学组成、键接方式、结构单元在空间排布的立体构型、支化和交联、共聚物的结构、高分子的大小和形态；以及高分子的远程结构，如高分子的结晶等。

（1）分子量与分子量分布　高分子之所以具有许多独特的性质，最重要的原因是其分子量大。这样高分子之间总的相互作用力就非常之大，所以高分子有很大的强度。分子量是评价高分子的重要指标。但高分子化合物的分子量是不均一的，实际上是一系列同系物的混合物，这种性质称为"多分散性"（polydispersity）。高分子的分子量一般都是指平均分子量，根据统计平均方法的不同，可以表示为数均分子量（$\bar{M}_n$）、重均分子质量（$\bar{M}_w$）等。高分子的多分散性可以用多分散指数（polydispersity index，PI）来定量表征，其定义为 $\bar{M}_w/\bar{M}_n$ 的比值。当分子量完全均一时，PI＝1；分子量分布越宽，比值越大。分子量分布也是影响高分子性能的重要因素。

（2）构型与构象　大分子链上结构单元中的取代基在空间上可能有的不同排布方式形成多种立体构型（configuration），主要有旋光异构和顺反异构两类。旋光异构由不对称碳原子引起；顺反异构是大分子链中的双键引起的。高分子链由于单键内旋转而产生的分子在空间的不同形态称为构象（conformation，又称内旋转异构体）。构象与构型的根本区别在于，构象通过单键内旋转可以改变，而构型无法通过内旋转改变。高分子的构象数非常多，因此高分子链由于内旋转能够不断改变其构象，这一性质称为柔顺性（简称柔性，flexibility）。这是高分子的许多性能不同于小分子物质的主要原因。

（3）高分子的形状和共聚物结构　一般高分子链为线型（称为线型高分子），也有支化、星形和交联等多种结构。交联高分子是一个三维空间网状大分子，不能熔融也不溶解，只能溶胀。如果高分子只有一种单体反应而成，称为均聚物；如果两种以上单体合成，则称为共聚物。以两种单体构成的二元共聚物为例，可能有无规共聚物、交替共聚物、嵌段共聚物和接枝共聚物四种序列结构。

（4）高分子的结晶性　高分子结晶结构通常是不完善的，有晶区也有非晶区。一根高分子链可以同时穿过晶区与非晶区。所以，结晶高分子不能100%结晶，其中总是存在非晶部分，实际上只能算半结晶高分子（semi-crystalline polymer）。非晶结构也称无定形结构，高分子大量存在的是非晶态结构。高分子的结晶度显著地影响着材料的性能，主要是力学性能和光学性能。

三、高分子的合成

除了自然界存在的天然高分子，我们现在使用的大多数高分子材料都是通过单体的聚合反应或者对现有高分子材料的改造获得的。聚合反应主要有两种类型，加聚反应（链式聚合）和缩聚反应（逐步聚合）。

烯类单体的加聚反应绝大多时属于链式聚合反应，一般由链增长、链引发、链终止等基元反应组成。聚合时引发剂先形成活性种 R*，活性种打开单体的 π 键，与之加成形成单体活性种，而后进一步不断与单体加成，促使链增长。最后，增长着的活性中心失去活性，使链终止。根据链增长活性中心的种类不同，可以分为自由基聚合、阴离子聚合、阳离子型聚合。以自由基聚合为例，引发剂分子能在较低的温度下分解产生自由基，很快同体系中的烯烃分子发生作用，使 π 键打开生成单体自由基，接着单体分子一个一个加成上去，自由基变得越来越长，直到最后遇到另一个自由基，相互合并在一起，变成一个稳定的大分子为止，这种终止形式称为偶合终止。链自由基还可能夺取另一自由基的氢原子或其他原子发生的链终止反应，称为岐化终止。而对于阴离子聚合，在无杂质存在的条件下，没有链终止反应，因为两个阴离子只会互相排斥，不可能结合在一起。若不外加终止剂，链活性中心直至全部单体消耗完仍能保持活性。如果向体系中再加入单体，这些单体会在高分子活性链末端继续生长，形成更高聚合度的高分子。这属于"活性聚合"（living polymerization）。活性聚合的特点是产物分子量分布非常窄，聚合产物的分子量与转化率成线性关系。因此，通过准确计算投料单体与引发剂的量，可以预期产物的聚合度。近年来，高分子科学家开发了原子转移自由基聚合（ATRP）、可逆加成-断裂链转移自由基聚合（RAFT）等多种新型的活性自由基聚合反应。

逐步聚合反应中，单体自身含有两个可以反应的基团，单体分子通过反复加成，在分子间形成共价键，逐步生成高分子量聚合物，同时可能伴随有小分子化合物的生成，如 H_2O、HCl、ROH 等。逐步聚合反应最重要的特征是，聚合体系中任何两分子（包括单体分子或聚合物分子）间都能相互反应生成聚合度更高的聚合物分子。聚合反应早期，单体很快消失，转变成低聚物，转化率已经很高而分子量却很低；而后的缩聚反应则在低聚物之间进行，延长聚合时间主要目的在于提高产物分子量，而不能提高转化率。

四、高分子的性能

（1）高分子的热性能　　高分子根据所处温度的不同，可能有 3 种不同的力学状态。在较低温度下，高分子的力学性质和玻璃差不多，弹性模量大，质硬，受力后形变很小，称为玻璃态。此时高分子的热运动能量低，链段处于被"冻结"的状态，只有侧基、链节、短支链等小运动单元的局部振动以及键长、键角的变化。随着温度的升高，链段开始"解冻"，虽然整个高分子链还不能移动，链分子可以在外力作用下伸展或卷曲。这种状态下的高分子弹性模量小，受较小外力即可产生很大形变，且形变是可逆的，处于高弹态。温度进一步升高，高分子链的热运动加剧，高分子开始呈现流动性，称为黏流态。其中，高分子由玻璃态向高弹态转变的温度称为玻璃化转变温度（T_g）。严格来说，T_g 是一个温度范围。在这个温度以上，高聚物表现为软而有弹性；在这个温度以下，高聚物则表现为硬而脆。

（2）高分子的力学性能　　高分子作为材料使用必须具有所需要的力学强度，主要指其在受力作用下产生形变以及抗破损的性能，可以通过测量应力-应变曲线、模量、强度、硬度等体现。高分子力学性能的最大特点是高弹性和黏弹性。高弹性的特点表现为弹性模量小、形变大；形变时伴随有热效应发生，伸长时放热，回缩时吸热。高分子在外力作用下发生变形是由于高分子链被伸展的结果，链伸展引起链构象数减少，熵值下降；热运动可使高分子链恢复到熵值最大、构象数最多的卷曲状态，因而产生弹性回复力，这就是弹性形变的本质。黏弹性指高分子不仅具有弹性而且有黏性，因为其形变的发展强烈依赖于温度和时间。这种力学性质随时间变化的现象称为力学松弛现象或黏弹性（viscoelasticity）现象。

五、高分子的表征技术

（1）分子量的测定　　凝胶渗透色谱（gel permeation chromatograghy, GPC），是常用的高分子分子量测定方法，它是一种利用多孔填料柱将溶液中的高分子按尺寸大小分离的色谱技术。分子尺寸较大的高分子渗透进入多孔填料孔洞中的几率较小，保留时间较短；尺寸较小的高分子则容易进入填料孔洞而且滞留时间较长。由此得出高分子尺寸大小随保留时间（或保留体积）变化的曲线，即分子量分布的色谱图。然后利用已知分子量高分子的标定曲线即可求出样品的重均分子量、数均分子量以及多分散系数。除此以外，测定高分子分子量的其他方法还有：端基分析法、黏度法、小角激光光散射法等。

（2）结构表征　高分子的化学结构可通过红外光谱、核磁进行表征。高分子的结晶情况可用 X 射线衍射法测定。

（3）示差扫描量热法　示差扫描量热法（differential scanning calorimetry，DSC）是用于研究高分子的热转变如玻璃化转变行为、熔融行为和结晶动态等的常用方法。其原理是在相同的程控温度变化下，用补偿器测量样品与参比物之间的温差保持为零所需热量对温度 T 的依赖关系。

六、高分子的加工

高分子材料的加工多数都是在液态下进行的，即用熔体或溶液加工，如注射成型、挤出成型、热压模塑、吹塑成型、纺丝等。少数是用固体粉末烧结成型，也有少数用单体或预聚物浇注成型或反应成型。高分子制品的性质不仅决定于原材料和配方，而且与加工方法密切相关。

References

[1] He P. Structure and Properties of Polymers. Alpha Science International Ltd, 2014.

[2] Cowie J M G, Arrighi A. Polymers: Chemistry and Physics of Modern Materials. 3rd Ed. CRC Press, 2008.

[3] Cooper s L, Visser S A, Hergenrother R W. Polymers, // B. Ratner, et al., Editors, Biomaterials Science: An Introduction to Materials in Medicine. Academic Press, 2004.

Chapter 3.

Natural Polymers as Pharmaceutical Excipients
天然来源的药用高分子辅料

3.1 Starch and its derivates

3.1.1 Starch

(1) Polymer description   Starch (amylum) is a kind of natural polysaccharide produced by green plants as an energy store. It is contained in large amounts of plants like potato, wheat, maize (corn), rice and tapioca, where starch molecules arrange themselves in semi-crystalline granules.

Structurally, starch is polysaccharide consisting of a large number of α-D-glucose units joined by glycosidic bonds. There are two types of starch molecules as shown in Figure 3-1, respectively: the linear and helical amylose and the branched amylopectin.

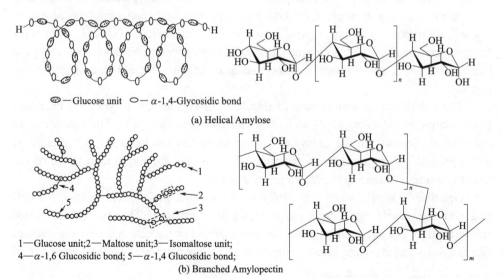

⬭—Glucose unit   ⬯— α-1,4-Glycosidic bond

(a) Helical Amylose

1—Glucose unit; 2—Maltose unit; 3—Isomaltose unit;
4—α-1,6 Glucosidic bond; 5—α-1,4 Glucosidic bond;

(b) Branched Amylopectin

Figure 3-1. Conformation and Structural formula of starch

Generally, starch contains 20%~25% amylose and 75%~80% amylopectin by weight. The anylose/amylopectin ratio differs depending on the plant source. For example, corn starch contains about 27% amylose, potato starch about 22%, and tapioca starch about 17%. Therefore, the physical properties of starches vary accordingly by these differences[1] so that the various types of starch may not be interchangeable in a given pharmaceutical application. Starch used in pharmaceuticals should be produced from corn, potato or wheat specified by the USPNF❶ XVII.

(2) Typical properties Pure starch occurs as an odorless and tasteless, white-colored powder comprised of very small spherical or ovoid granules whose size and shape are characteristic for each botanical variety. All starches are hygroscopic and rapidly absorb atmospheric moisture. Commercially available grades of corn starch usually contain 10%~14% water.

① *Solubility* Starch is insoluble in cold water or alcohol, which swells instantaneously in water by about 5%~10% at 37℃.

② *Gelatinization of starch* When starch is heated in water, the granules swell and burst, forming a network that holds water and increasing the mixture's viscosity. This process is called starch gelatinization. Gelatinization is a process that breaks down the intermolecular bonds of starch molecules in the presence of water and heat, allowing the hydrogen bonding sites (the hydroxyl hydrogen and oxygen) to engage more water. During gelatinization of starch, three main processes happen to the starch granule: granule swelling, crystal or double helical melting, and amylose leaching. Water is first absorbed in the amorphous space of starch which leads to a swelling phenomenon during heating, and then transmits through connecting molecules to crystalline regions, causing crystalline structures to melt and break free. This irreversibly dissolves the starch granule. Penetration of water increases randomness in the general starch granule structure and decreases the number and size of crystalline regions.

The gelatinization temperature of starch depends upon plant type. For example, potato starch start swelling at 56~66℃, and maize starch at 62~72℃. The gelatinization temperature depends on the cross-linking degree of the amylopectin. The amount of water present, pH, types and concentration of salt, sugar, fat and protein in the recipe are also factors influencing the starch gelatinization.

Gelatinized starch, when cooled for a long enough period, will thicken (or gel) and rearrange itself again to a more crystalline structure. This process is called retrogradation. During cooling, molecular associations occur between starch molecules like amylose-amylose, amylose-amylopectin or amylopectin-amylopectin. It is a mild

---

❶ USP-NF is a combination of two compendia, the United States Pharmacopeia (USP) and the National Formulary (NF). It contains public pharmacopeial standards. Monographs for drug substances, dosage forms, and compounded preparations are featured in the USP. Monographs for dietary supplements and ingredients appear in a separate section of the USP. Excipient monographs are in the NF.

association amongst chains together with water still embedded in the molecule. Due to the tightly packed organization of small granule starches, retrogradation occurs much more slowly compared to larger starch granules. Due to strong associations of hydrogen bonding, longer amylose molecules will form a stiff gel. Amylopectin molecules with longer branched structure increase the tendency to form strong gels. High amylopectin starches will have a stable gel, but will be softer than high amylose gels. Retrogradation restricts the availability for amylase hydrolysis to occur.

③ *Stability and storage conditions* Dry and unheated starch is stable if protected from high humidity. Starch should be stored in an airtight container in a cool and dry place. However, heated starch solutions or pastes are physically unstable and are readily attacked by microorganisms to form a wide variety of starch derivatives.

④ *Safety* Starch is generally regarded as an essentially nontoxic and nonirritant material. It is GRAS❶ listed and included in the FDA Inactive Ingredients Guide. It is also included in nonparenteral medicines licensed in the UK. However, oral consumption of massive doses can be harmful due to the formation of starch calculi which cause bowel obstruction. Lethal dose 50% (LD_{50}) of starch is 6.6g/kg determined in mouse by intraperitoneal injection (IP). The application of starch to the peritoneum or the meninges or surgical wounds may cause granulomatous reactions. Allergic reactions to starch are extremely rare.

(3) Applications in pharmaceutical formulation or technology Starch is widely used as an excipient primarily in oral solid dosage formulations where it is utilized as a binder, diluent or disintegrant.

In tablet formulations, freshly prepared starch paste is used at a concentration of 5%~25% (*w/w*) in tablet granulations as a binder. Selection of the quantity required in a given system is determined by optimization studies, using parameters such as granule friability, tablet friability, hardness, disintegration rate and drug dissolution rate.

As a diluent, starch is used for the preparation of standardized triturates of colorants or potent drugs to facilitate subsequent mixing or blending processes in manufacturing operations. Starch is also used in dry-filled capsule formulations for volume adjustment of the fill matrix.

Starch is one of the most commonly used tablet disintegrants at concentrations of 3%~15% (*w/w*). However, unmodified starch does not compress well and tends to increase tablet friability if used in high concentrations. In granulated formulations, about half of the total starch content is included in the granulation mixture and the balance is added as part of the final blend with the dried granulation.

Starch is also used in topical preparations. For example, it is widely used in

---

❶ "GRAS" is an acronym for the phrase "generally recognized as safe". Generally recognized as safe (GRAS) is an American Food and Drug Administration (FDA) designation that a chemical or substance added to food is considered safe by experts, and so is exempted from the usual Federal Food, Drug, and Cosmetic Act (FFDCA) food additive tolerance requirements.

dusting-powders for its absorbency, and is used as a protective covering in ointment formulations applied to the skin. Starch mucilage has also been applied to the skin as an emollient. Starch mucilage has formed the base of some enemas for use in the treatment of iodine poisoning.

Therapeutically, rice starch based solutions have been used in the prevention and treatment of dehydration due to acute diarrheal diseases.

3.1.2 Pregelatinized starch

(1) Polymer description   Pregelatinized starch is a starch that has been chemically and mechanically processed to rupture all or part of the starch granules, which renders the starch flowable and directly compressible as results. The difference in morphology between pregelatinized starch and natural maize starch is shown in Figure 3-2. Typically, pregelatinized starch contains 5% of free amylose, 15% of free amylopectin and 80% of unmodified starch. Partially pregelatinized grades are also commercially available.

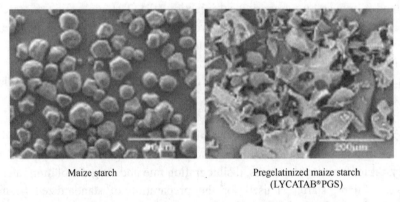

Maize starch   Pregelatinized maize starch
                                    (LYCATAB®PGS)

Figure 3-2. SEM images of maize starch and pregelatinized maize starch.

Fully pregelatinized starch is prepared by heating an aqueous slurry containing up to 42% (w/w) of starch at 62~72°C. Gelatinization aids (salts or bases) and surfactants may be added in the slurry to control rehydration or minimize stickiness during drying. After heating, the slurry may be spray-dried, roll-dried, extruded or drum-dried. In the latter case, the dried material may be processed to produce a desired particle size range.

Partially pregelatinized starch is prepared by spreading an aqueous suspension of ungelatinized starch on hot drums where partial gelatinization and subsequent drying takes place.

(2) Typical properties   Pregelatinized starch occurs as white to off-white colored powder, which is odorless and has a slight characteristic taste. Pregelatinized maize starch is hygroscopic.

① *Solubility*   Pregelatinized starch is practically insoluble in organic solvents. It is lightly soluble in cold water, depending upon the degree of pregelatinization. Fully pregelatinized starch is soluble.

② *Stability and storage conditions*   Pregelatinized starch is stable but hygroscopic, which should be stored in a well-closed container in a cool and dry place.

③ *Safety*   Similar as starch.

(3) Applications in pharmaceutical formulation or technology   Pregelatinized starch is usually used in oral capsule and tablet formulations as a binder, diluent and disintegrant.

In comparison to starch, the pregelatinized starch shows enhanced flow and compression characteristics, so it may be used as a tablet binder in dry compression processes. In such processes, pregelatinized starch is self-lubricating. However, it is necessary to add a lubricant to a formulation when pregelatinized starch is used with other excipients. Stearic acid is generally the preferred lubricant with pregelatinized starch. Pregelatinized starch may also be used in wet granulation processes.

Starch 1500, a partially pregelatinized maize starch produced by Colorcon Ltd, is a unique pharmaceutical excipient combining several properties in a single product: binder, disintegrant, filler and flow-aid while having lubricant properties. It is particularly effective with moisture sensitive actives and low dose applications. In addition to providing a unique range of functions and flexible performance in a variety of applications, Starch 1500 cuts process and material costs by reducing or eliminating polymeric binders, superdisintegrants, high levels of lubricants and glidants and manufacturing steps.

Starch 1500 L.M. (Colorcon Ltd) is a low moisture grade of pregelatinized starch, containing less than 7% of water. It is commercially available specifically intended for use as a diluent in capsule formulations.

LYCATAB® PGS is a pregelatinized maize starch that has been specially developed as a robust binder for wet granulation. It is dispersible in cold water and ready for use. LYCATAB® C, another product of partially pregelatinized starch, is a suitable ingredient for direct compression tableting and capsule filling. It is a multipurpose excipient combining the dilution and disintegration power of native starch with flowability and controlled cohesive power.

3.1.3   Dextrin

(1) Polymer description   Dextrin is partially hydrolyzed starch with molecular weight in 4500~85000 typically. The BP[❶] 1993 specifies that dextrin is derived from

---

❶ British Pharmacopoeia (BP): a publication of the General Medical Council (UK) describing and establishing standards for medicines, preparations, materials and articles used in the practice of medicine, surgery and midwifery. The first British Pharmacopoeia was published in 1864.

maize or potato starch.

Dextrin is prepared by the incomplete hydrolysis of starch by heating in the dry state with or without the aid of suitable acids and buffers. This process is known as dextrinization. Dextrins are mainly yellow to brown in color and dextrinization is partially responsible for the browning of toasted bread.

Normally, the available dextrin from suppliers is in a number of modified forms and mixtures such as dextri-maltose. Dextri-maltose is a mixture of maltose and dextrin obtained by the enzymatic action of barley malt on corn flour. It is a light amorphous powder, readily soluble in milk or water.

(2) Typical properties   Dextrin is a white, pale yellow or brown-colored powder with a slight characteristic odor.

① *Solubility*   Dextrin is slowly soluble in water and it is very soluble in boiling water forming a mucilaginous solution. Dextrin is practically insoluble in chloroform, ethanol (95%), ether and propan-2-ol.

② *Stability and storage conditions*   Dry dextrin is stable, but incompatible with strong oxidizing agents. The bulk material should be stored in a well-closed container in a cool and dry place. In aqueous solutions, dextrin molecules tend to aggregate as density, temperature, pH, or other characteristics change. An increase in viscosity is caused by gelation or retrogradation as dextrin solutions age. Dextrin solutions are thixotropic, becoming less viscous when sheared but changing to a soft paste or gel when allowed to stand. However, acids that are present in dextrin as residues from manufacturing will cause further hydrolysis which results in a gradual thinning of solutions. Residual acid will also cause a reduction in viscosity during dry storage. To eliminate these problems, dextrin manufacturers usually neutralize dextrins of low solubility with ammonia or sodium carbonate in the cooling vessel.

③*Safety*   Dextrin is generally regarded as a nontoxic and nonirritant material at the levels employed as an excipient. Although ingestion of very large quantities may be harmful, larger quantities of dextrin are used as a dietary supplement without adverse effects.

(3) Applications in pharmaceutical formulation or technology   Dextrin is usually used as diluents in a tablet and capsule, a binder for tablet granulation and a thickening agent for suspensions. It is also utilized as a sugar coating ingredient, which serves as a plasticizer and adhesive.

It was reported that starch-dextrin mixtures are used as principal excipients for extrusion-spheronization pellets with the aim of producing pellets with more suitable properties for certain types of release [2]. Results show that the mixtures of notably starch (corn starch or wheat starch) and 20% white dextrin gave high-quality pellets with good size and shape distributions.

3.1.4 Cyclodextrin

(1) Polymer description   Cyclodextrins are cyclic oligosaccharides derived from starch, which contain at least 6 D-(+)-glucopyranose units attached by α-(1→4) glucoside bonds in a ring, creating a cone shape. There are three natural cyclodextrins, α, β, and γ, containing 6, 7 and 8 glucopyranose units respectively. They thus have a rigid structure with a central cavity whose size varies according to the cyclodextrin type. Scheme 3-1 shows the structural formula of β-cyclodextrin and its derivates.

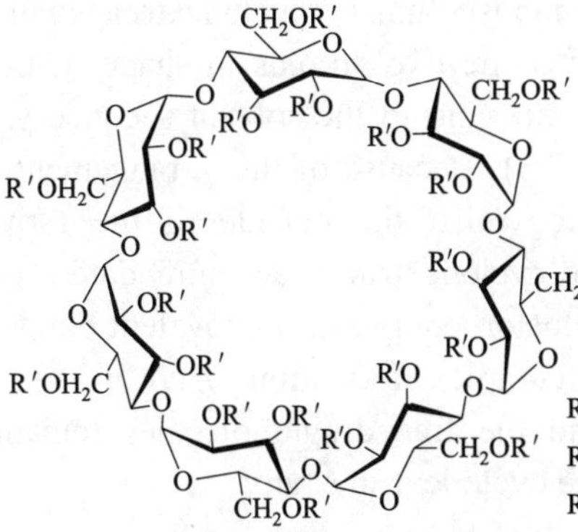

R′, R″=–H for β-cyclodextrin (7 glucose units)
R′, R″=–CHOHCH₃ for hydroxyethyl- β-cyclodextrin
R′, R″=–CH₂CHOHCH₃ for hydroxypropyl- β-cyclodextrin

Scheme 3-1. Structural formula of β-cyclodextrin and its derivates.

Cyclodextrins containing 9, 10, 11, 12 and 13 glucopyranose units have also been reported. Though hundreds of modified cyclodextrins have been prepared and shown to have research applications, only a few of these derivatives containing the hydroxypropyl (HP), methyl (M) and sulfobutylether (SBE) substituents have been commercially used as new pharmaceutical excipients.

Cyclodextrins are manufactured by the enzymatic degradation of starch using specialized bacteria. An organic solvent is used to direct the reaction to produce β-cyclodextrin and to prevent the growth of microorganisms during the enzymatic reaction. The insoluble β-cyclodextrin organic solvent complex is separated from the non-cyclic starch, and the organic solvent is removed in vacuum. The β-cyclodextrin is then carbon treated and crystallized from water, dried, and collected. Hydroxyethyl-β-cyclodextrin is made by reacting β-cyclodextrin with ethylene oxide, whilst hydroxypropyl-β-cyclodextrin is made by reacting β-cyclodextrin with propylene oxide.

(2) Typical Properties   Cyclodextrins occur as white, practically odorless, fine crystalline powders, having a slightly sweet taste. Some cyclodextrin derivatives occur as amorphous powders.

① *Solubility*   Solubility of cyclodextrins varies a little depending on the different type as shown in Table 3-1.

Table 3-1. Solubility of different cyclodextrins.

Type of cyclodextrin	Solubility
α-cyclodextrin	soluble 1 in 7 parts of water at 20℃, 1 in 3 at 50℃.
β-cyclodextrin	soluble 1 in 200 parts of propylene glycol;
	soluble 1 in 50 parts of water at 20℃, 1 in 20 at 50℃;
	insoluble in acetone and ethanol (95%)
γ-cyclodextrin	soluble 1 in 4.4 parts of water at 20℃, 1 in 2 at 45℃

② *Cyclodextrin inclusion complexation* Owing to the lack of free rotation around the bonds connecting the glucopyranose units, cyclodextrins can be topologically represented as 'bucket-like' or 'cone-like' toroids in shape, with the larger and the smaller openings of the toroid exposing to the solvent secondary and primary hydroxyl groups respectively (Figure 3-3). Because of this arrangement, the internal surface of the cavity is hydrophobic whilst the outside of the torus is hydrophilic. This arrangement thus permits the cyclodextrin to accommodate a guest molecule within the host cavity to form an inclusion complex. No covalent bonds are formed or broken during drug-cyclodextrin complex formation. And in aqueous solution, the complexes readily dissociate and the free drug molecules remain in equilibrium with the molecules bound within the cyclodextrin cavity.

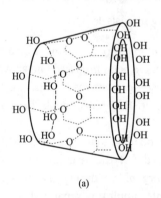
(a)

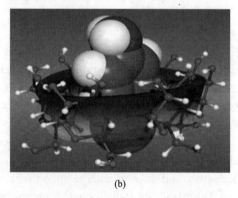
(b)

Figure 3-3. (a) Toroid structure of γ-Cyclodextrin showing spatial arrangement.
(b) Schematic diagram of host & guest molecular interaction.

③ *Stability and storage conditions* β-cyclodextrin and other cyclodextrins, are stable in the solid state if protected from high humidity. They should be stored in a tightly sealed container in a cool and dry place.

④ *Safety* Cyclodextrins are generally regarded as essentially nontoxic and nonirritant materials. They are not irritant to the skin and eyes, or upon inhalation. Cyclodextrin administered orally is metabolized by microflora in the colon forming the metabolites maltodextrin, maltose and glucose, which are further metabolized and excreted as carbon dioxide and water. Therefore, cyclodextrins are now approved for use in food products and orally administered pharmaceuticals in a number of countries. However, when parenterally administered, β-cyclodextrin is not metabolized but accumulates in the kidneys as insoluble cholesterol complexes, resulting in severe nephrotoxicity. Neither is there any evidence to suggest that cyclodextrins are mutagenic or teratogenic.

⑤ *Incompatibility* The activity of some antimicrobial preservatives in aqueous solution can be reduced in the presence of hydroxypropyl-β-cyclodextrin.

(3) Applications in pharmaceutical formulation or technology In the pharmaceutical industry cyclodextrins have mainly been used as complexing agents to increase aqueous solubility of poorly soluble drugs, and to increase their bioavailability and stability. Table 3-2 exhibits the solubility of different drugs in water and in 50% 2-HP-β-cyclodextrin. Moreover, cyclodextrin inclusion complexes in formulations may help mask the unpleasant taste of active materials, reduce the drug induced irritation and convert a liquid substance into a solid material. For example, an itraconazole oral preparation contains 40% (*w/v*) of HP-β-cyclodextrin. Currently there are approximately 30 different pharmaceutical products worldwide containing drug/cyclodextrin complexes on the market[3, 4].

Table 3-2. Solubility (25℃) of drugs in water and 2-HP-β-Cyclodextrin.

Drug	Solubility in water /(g/L)	Solubility in 50% 2-HP-β-yclodextrin /(g/L)
Vitamin A	0.001	4.6
Dexamethasone	0.008	44.3
17-β-Estradiol	0.004	40.5
Methotrexate	0.045	10.0
Norethisterone	0.005	19.0
Progesterone	0.002	4.9
Phenytoin	0.02	9.3

β-Cyclodextrin is the most commonly used cyclodextrin although it is the least soluble. β-Cyclodextrin has been primarily used in tablet and capsule formulations. In oral tablet formulations β-cyclodextrin may be used in both wet granulation and direct compression processes. Whilst the physical properties of β-cyclodextrin vary from manufacturer to manufacturer, β-cyclodextrin tends to possess poor flow properties and requires a lubricant, such as 0.1% (*w/w*) magnesium stearate, when it is directly compressed.

α-Cyclodextrin is mainly used in parenteral formulations, although it can only form inclusion complexes with relatively few and small sized molecules due to the smallest cavity of the cyclodextrins. In contrast, γ-cyclodextrin has the largest cavity and can be used to form inclusion complexes with large molecules, which may also be used in parenteral formulations.

3.1.5 Sodium carboxymethyl starch

(1) Polymer description Structural formula of sodium carboxymethyl starch:

R=CH₂COONa—, H

Sodium carboxymethyl starch (also named as sodium starch glycolate) is the sodium salt of a carboxymethyl ether of starch. It is prepared by reacting starch with sodium chloroacetate in an alkaline medium followed by neutralization with citric, or some other acid. Sodium carboxymethyl starch may be characterized by the degree of substitution. The molecular weight is typically 500000~1000000.

(2) Typical properties Sodium carboxymethyl starch is a white to off-white, odorless, tasteless, and free-flowing powder. It consists of oval or spherical granules, 30~100μm in diameter, with some less-spherical granules ranging in 10~35μm in diameter.

① *Solubility and swelling capacity* Sodium carboxymethyl starch is sparingly soluble in ethanol (95%) and practically insoluble in water. But it can swell with its volume increased up to 300 times in water. At a concentration of 2% (*w/v*), sodium carboxymethyl starch disperses in cold water and settles in the form of a highly hydrated layer.

② *Stability and storage conditions* Sodium carboxymethyl starch is stable and should be stored in a well-closed container to protect it from wide variations in humidity and temperature. The physical properties of sodium carboxymethyl starch remain unchanged for up to four years if stored at moderate temperatures and humidity.

③ *Safety* Sodium carboxymethyl starch is generally regarded as a nontoxic and nonirritant material. However, oral ingestion of large quantities may be harmful.

(3) Applications in pharmaceutical formulation or technology Sodium carboxymethyl starch is widely used in oral pharmaceuticals as a disintegrant in capsule and tablet formulations. It is commonly used in tablets prepared by either direct compression or wet granulation processes. The usual concentration employed in a formulation is between 2%~8%, with the optimum concentration about 4% although in many cases 2% is sufficient. Disintegration occurs by rapid uptake of water followed by rapid and enormous swelling. It is noted that the disintegrant efficiency of sodium carboxymethyl starch is unimpaired by the presence of hydrophobic excipients, such as lubricants. And increasing the tablet compression pressure also appears to have no effect on disintegration time.

GLYCOLYS® (Figure 3-4) is a superdisintegrant produced by Roquette, which exhibits the superdisintegration function in solid dosage forms like tablets and capsules.

The usual recommended concentration is 2%~4%, however the optimum quantity to be used in a formulation should be experimentally determined. Roquette has been developing different grades of GLYCOLYS® sodium carboxymethyl starch to meet particular needs, eg. viscosity, pH or solvent-free properties. For example, GLYCOLYS® Low pH grade is specifically designed to resist acidic pH and maintain stability in formulations containing strongly acidic drugs.

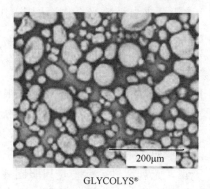

GLYCOLYS®

Figure 3-4. SEM image of GLYCOLYS® sodium carboxymethyl starch.

◆ 本节中文导读 ◆

淀粉及其衍生物是指天然淀粉及由天然淀粉经物理或化学改性制备的产物，它们是医药工业和食品工业应用最多的天然高分子。

（1）淀粉（starch） 淀粉是来自植物光合作用形成的以 α-D-葡萄糖为结构单元的高分子量多糖，通常为无臭、无味球状或卵形颗粒状白色粉末。药用淀粉多为玉米淀粉、马铃薯淀粉和小麦淀粉。淀粉经热水处理，约有 25%能溶解，可溶部分称为直链淀粉，其余 75％为不溶部分，称支链淀粉。淀粉具有微弱亲水性并能分散于水，淀粉不溶于水、乙醇和乙醚等，但吸湿性很强，能迅速吸收空气中的水分。市售淀粉一般含水分 10%～14%。淀粉在水中加热至 60～80℃时，颗粒可逆地吸水膨胀，至某一温度时整个颗粒突然大量膨化、破裂，晶体结构消失，最终变成均匀黏稠的糊，这种现象称为淀粉的糊化，发生糊化所需的温度成为糊化温度。 淀粉可食用，无毒、无刺激性。淀粉是口服固体制剂的基本辅料，在制粒中用作胶黏剂，在生产中后续混合操作用作稀释剂，在片剂的制备中用作崩解剂。淀粉用于局部用制剂，在软膏制剂中起到皮肤覆盖层的作用。淀粉胶浆可用做润肤剂，用来制备灌肠剂的基料，用来处置碘中毒。

（2）预胶化淀粉（pregelatinized starch） 预胶化淀粉是用化学法或机械法将淀粉颗粒部分或全部破裂的产物，为白色或类白色、无臭、微有特殊口感的粉末。预胶化淀粉稳定但容易吸湿，不溶于有机溶剂，微溶以至可溶于冷水，具有良好的流动性、直接可压性、自身润滑性和干黏合性，并有较好的崩解作用。作为多功能辅料，预胶化淀粉广泛用于口服固体药物制剂中，作为片剂和胶囊剂的稀释剂、片剂和胶囊剂的崩解剂、片剂的胶黏剂和色素的展延剂等。与淀粉相比，预胶化淀粉能增加流动性和可压性。由于游离态支链淀粉润湿后的巨大溶胀作用和非游离态部分的变形复原作用，预胶化淀粉具有良好的促进崩解作用且崩解作用不受崩解液 pH 的影响。

（3）糊精（dextrin） 糊精为玉米或马铃薯淀粉水解产物，无毒，无刺激性。糊精几乎不溶于氯仿、95％乙醇、乙醚和丙二醇，缓慢溶解于冷水，极易溶于沸水并形成胶浆状溶液。糊精溶液具有触变性，剪切作用下黏度降低，静置后成糊或成凝胶。糊精可用作外科手术敷料的胶黏剂和硬化剂，片剂和胶囊剂的稀释剂，片剂颗粒的胶黏剂，糖包衣配方中的增塑剂和胶黏剂，或混悬剂的增稠剂。

（4）环糊精（cyclodextrins） 环糊精是用环糊精葡糖基转移酶作用于淀粉或淀粉水解产物而得的淀粉衍生物。环糊精结构为环状寡聚糖，由 α（1→4）苷键连接的 D-(+)-吡喃葡萄糖单元组成。α-、β-和 γ-环糊精分别含有 6、7 和 8 个葡萄糖单元，不同种类的环糊精，其溶解性、密度、熔点、含水量等基本性质略有差别。环糊精分子是由刚性结构及中心空腔构成的"桶状"环形分子，空腔内表面具有疏水性，外部具有亲水性，空腔大小根据环糊精类型不同而不同。因此，环糊精可以在空腔内容纳客体分子，制备药物分子的包合物，从而增加药物溶解度、提高药物的化学和物理稳定性。环糊精包合物还可用来掩盖活性物质的不良味道，将液体物质转化为固体材料。

（5）羧甲淀粉钠（sodium starch glycolate） 羧甲淀粉钠淀粉的羧甲醚钠盐，分子量一般在 $5×10^5～1×10^6$。羧甲淀粉钠微溶于乙醇(95%)；几乎不溶于水，可以 2%（质量浓度）的浓度分散在水中，静置时形成高度水化的溶胀层。羧甲淀粉钠很稳定，用羧甲淀粉钠制得的片剂具有良好的贮藏性质。羧甲淀粉钠在水中可快速溶胀达自身原体积的 300 倍，作为一种性能优良的崩解剂广泛应用于口服药物制剂中，如用于直接压片或湿法制粒的片剂中，最佳用量约为 4%。羧甲淀粉钠还可用作助悬剂。

3.2　Cellulose and its derivates

Cellulose is a polysaccharide consisting of a linear chain of several hundreds to over ten thousands $\beta(1\rightarrow4)$ linked D-glucose units, with the structural formula as shown below. Cellulose is an important structural component of the primary cell wall of green plants. The cellulose content of cotton fiber is 90%, that of wood is 40%~50% and that of dried hemp is approximately 45%. Cellulose is the most abundant natural polymer on the earth.

Structural formula of cellulose:

Cellulose is a straight chain polymer. It should be noted that D-glucose units condense through $\beta(1\rightarrow4)$-glycosidic bonds in cellulose, contrasting with $\alpha(1\rightarrow4)$-glycosidic bonds present in starch. Thus, the molecule of cellulose adopts an extended and rather stiff rod-like conformation, aided by the equatorial conformation of the glucose residues. The multiple hydroxyl groups on the glucose from one chain form hydrogen bonds with oxygen atoms on the same or on a neighbor chain, holding the chains firmly together side-by-side and forming microfibrils with high tensile strength. Therefore, cellulose is much more crystalline, compared to starch.

Generally, cellulose has no taste and is odorless. It is hydrophilic with the contact angle of $20°\sim30°$, but is insoluble in water and most organic solvents. Cellulose is biodegradable. It can be broken down chemically into its glucose units by treating it with concentrated acids at high temperature.

The hydroxyl groups of cellulose can be partially or fully reacted with various reagents to afford derivatives with useful properties like mainly cellulose esters and cellulose ethers. The excipients used in pharmaceutics include a variety of cellulose derivatives.

3.2.1　Microcrystalline cellulose

(1) Polymer description　Microcrystalline cellulose is a kind of purified and partially depolymerized cellulose, which is manufactured by the controlled hydrolysis of α-cellulose (obtained as a pulp from fibrous plant materials) with dilute mineral acid solutions. Following hydrolysis, the hydrocellulose is purified by filtration and the aqueous slurry is spray-dried to form dry and porous particles of a broad size

distribution.

Microcrystalline cellulose is commercially available in different particle size grades with different properties and applications. The typical mean particle size is 20~200 μm.

(2) Typical properties　Microcrystalline cellulose occurs as a white-colored, odorless, tasteless and crystalline powder composed of porous particles. Microcrystalline cellulose is hygroscopic. The moisture content is typically less than 5% *w/w*.

① *Solubility*　Microcrystalline cellulose is slightly soluble in 5% (*w/v*) sodium hydroxide solution and is practically insoluble in water, dilute acids and most organic solvents.

② *Stability and storage conditions*　Microcrystalline cellulose is stable, but is incompatible with strong oxidizing agents. The bulk material should be stored in a well-closed container in a cool and dry place.

③ *Safety*　Microcrystalline cellulose is generally regarded as a nontoxic and nonirritant material following oral administration. However, consumption of large quantities of cellulose may have a laxative effect. Deliberate abuse of formulations containing cellulose, either by inhalation or injection, has resulted in the formation of cellulose granulomas.

(3) Applications in pharmaceutical formulation or technology　Microcrystalline cellulose is widely used in pharmaceuticals as a diluent in oral tablet and capsule formulations. It can be used in both wet granulation and direct compression processes. In addition, microcrystalline cellulose also has some lubricant and disintegrant properties when used in tablet.

3.2.2　Powdered cellulose

(1) Polymer description　Powdered cellulose is manufactured by the purification and mechanical size reduction of α-cellulose. Different grades of powdered cellulose are commercially available in several different particle sizes, which range from a free-flowing fine or granular dense powder to a coarse, fluffy and non-flowing material.

(2) Typical properties　Powdered cellulose occurs as a white or almost white, odorless and tasteless powder of various particle sizes. Powdered cellulose is slightly hygroscopic.

① *Solubility*　Powdered cellulose disperses in most liquids, but is practically insoluble in water, dilute acids and most organic solvents. It is slightly soluble in 5% *w/v* sodium hydroxide solution. Powdered cellulose does not swell in water, but does in dilute bleach.

② *Safety*　Powdered cellulose is not absorbed systemically following oral administration and thus is generally regards as a nontoxic and nonirritant material.

(3) Applications in pharmaceutical formulation or technology   Powdered cellulose is used as a tablet diluent and a hard gelatin capsule filler. It has acceptable compression properties although its flow properties are poor. In soft gelatin capsules, powdered cellulose may be used to reduce the sedimentation of oily suspension fills.

Powdered cellulose is additionally used as the powder base material of powder dosage forms and as a suspending agent in aqueous suspensions for peroral delivery. It may also be used to reduce sedimentation during the manufacture of suppositories.

3.2.3 Methylcellulose

(1) Polymer description   *Structural formula of methylcellulose*:

Methylcellulose is a kind of substituted cellulose derivate in which approximately 27%~32% of the hydroxyl groups are in the form of the methyl ether. The degree of substitution of methylcellulose is defined as the average number of methoxyl (CH_3O—) groups attached to each of the anhydroglucose units along the chain, which affects the physical properties of methylcellulose, such as its solubility. Various grades of methylcellulose have different polymerization degree of anhydroglucose units in the range of 50~1500.

Methylcellulose is usually prepared from wood pulp by treatment with alkali followed by methylation of the alkali cellulose with chloromethane.

(2) Typical properties   Methylcellulose occurs as practically odorless and tasteless, white to yellowish-white colored granules or as a powder.

① *Solubility*   Methylcellulose is practically insoluble in acetone, chloroform, ethanol, ether, saturated salt solutions, toluene and hot water. It is soluble in glacial acetic acid and in a mixture of equal volumes of ethanol and chloroform. In cold water, methylcellulose swells and disperses slowly to form a clear to opalescent, viscous and colloidal dispersion.

The most commonly used method to dissolve methylcellulose is to add it initially to hot water. Firstly, the appropriate quantity of methylcellulose is mixed with about half the desired final volume of water at 70℃. Then cold or ice water is added to the hot methylcellulose slurry to cool it to below 20℃. A clear aqueous methylcellulose solution is thus obtained. Various grades of methylcellulose are commercially available which produce 2% (*w/v*) solutions with viscosities of 10~10000mPa • s. The viscosity of solutions may be increased by increasing the concentration of methylcellulose and reduced on heating until gel formation occurs at

$50 \sim 60 \,^{\circ}\mathrm{C}$. The process of thermogelation is reversible, with a viscous solution being reformed on cooling.

② *Stability and storage conditions*   Methylcellulose powder is stable with slight hygroscopicity. The bulk material should be stored in an airtight container in a cool and dry place.

Solutions of methylcellulose are stable to alkalis and dilute acids between pH=3~11 at room temperature. At less than pH=3, the viscosity of methylcellulose solutions is reduced. Methylcellulose solutions are liable to microbial spoilage and should be preserved with an antimicrobial preservative. Methylcellulose solutions may be sterilized by autoclaving. But this process can decrease the viscosity of a solution. Such change in viscosity is related to solution pH, where solutions at less than pH=4 have their viscosities reduced by more than 20%.

③ *Incompatibility*   Methylcellulose is reported to be incompatible with aminacrine hydrochloride, chlorocresol, mercuric chloride, phenol, resorcinol, tannic acid, silver nitrate, cetylpyridinium chloride, p-hydroxybenzoic acid, p-aminobenzoic acid: methylparaben, propylparaben and butylparaben. Complexation of methylcellulose occurs with highly surface-active compounds, such as tetracaine and dibutoline sulfate. High concentrations of electrolytes increase the viscosity of methylcellulose solutions inducing the salting out of methylcellulose. With very high concentrations of electrolytes, the methylcellulose may be completely precipitated in the form of a discrete or continuous gel.

④ *Safety*   Methylcellulose is generally regarded as a nontoxic, nonallergenic and nonirritant material. Methylcellulose is a noncaloric material, which is not digested or absorbed following oral consumption. Ingestion of excessive amounts of methylcellulose may temporarily increase flatulence and gastrointestinal distension. However, consumption of methylcellulose may aggravate obstructive gastrointestinal diseases in certain individuals. Oesophageal obstruction may also occur if methylcellulose is swallowed with an insufficient quantity of fluid. Moreover, consumption of large quantities of methylcellulose may additionally interfere with the normal absorption of some minerals. Methylcellulose is not commonly used in parenteral product although it has been used in intra-articular and intramuscular injections. Studies in rats have suggested that parenterally administered methylcellulose may cause glomerulonephritis and hypertension.

(3) Applications in pharmaceutical formulation or technology   Methylcellulose is widely used in oral and topical pharmaceutical formulations, as listed in Table 3-3.

Medium or high viscosity grades are used as bulk laxatives in the normal individual, in which oral consumption of large amounts of methylcellulose has a laxative action. The daily dose is about 1~6 g of methylcellulose in the form of granules or tablets, dividedly administered with plenty of fluid.

Table 3-3. The usage of methylcellulose in pharmaceutical formulations.

Usage	Concentration /%
Bulk laxative	5~30
Creams, gels and ointments	1~5
Emulsifying agent	1~5
Ophthalmic preparations	0.5~1.0
Suspensions	1~2
Sustained release tablet matrix	5~75
Tablet binder	2~6
Tablet coating	0.5~5
Tablet disintegrant	2~10

In tablet formulations, low or medium viscosity grades of methylcellulose are used as binding agents, which may be added either as a dry powder or in solution. High viscosity grades of methylcellulose may also be incorporated in tablet formulations as a disintegrant. Methylcellulose may also be added to a tablet formulation to produce sustained release preparations, where the methylcellulose is uniformly incorporated throughout a tablet in a hydrophilic matrix. Upon contact with water the outer tablet skin partially hydrates to form a gel layer. The overall dissolution rate is controlled by the erosion rate of this gel layer or diffusion of an active ingredient through it.

The aqueous or organic solutions of highly substituted and low viscosity grades of methylcellulose may also be used to spray-coat tablet cores in order to mask an unpleasant taste or to modify the release of a drug. Methylcellulose coats are used for sealing tablet cores prior to sugar coating.

Low viscosity grades of methylcellulose are used to emulsify olive, peanut and mineral oils. They are also used as suspending or thickening agents for orally administered liquids, commonly in place of sugar-based syrups or other suspension bases. The function of methylcellulose is to delay the settling of suspensions and to increase the contact time of drugs in the stomach.

High viscosity grades of methylcellulose are used to thicken topically applied products such as creams and gels.

In ophthalmic preparations, a 0.5%~1.0% (*w/v*) solution of a highly substituted and high viscosity grade of methylcellulose has been used as a vehicle for eye-drops. An antimicrobial preservative, such as benzalkonium chloride should also be included. However, hydroxypropyl methylcellulose based formulations are now preferred for ophthalmic preparations.

3.2.4　Ethylcellulose

(1) Polymer description　*Structural formula of ethylcellulose*:

n, R=CH$_3$CH$_2$—, H

Ethylcellulose is an ethyl ether of cellulose, which is prepared from wood pulp by treatment with alkali followed by ethylation of the alkali cellulose with chloroethane. Various grades of ethylcellulose are commercially available which differ in their ethoxyl content and degree of polymerization. Usually, the degree of substitution (DS) is about 2.25~2.60 ethoxyl groups (OC$_2$H$_5$) per anhydroglucose unit, equivalent to an ethoxyl content of 44%~51%.

(2) Typical properties   Ethylcellulose is a tasteless, free-flowing and white to light tan colored powder. The glass transition temperature (T_g) of ethylcellulose is at about 130~133℃. Ethylcellulose has poor hygroscopicity, which absorbs very little water at high relative humidities or during immersion.

① *Solubility*   Ethylcellulose is practically insoluble in glycerin, propylene glycol and water. The solubility of ethylcellulose varies depending on the ethoxyl content. Ethylcellulose that contains less than 46.5% ethoxyl groups is freely soluble in chloroform, methyl acetate, tetrahydrofuran, and in mixtures of aromatic hydrocarbons with ethanol (95%). Ethylcellulose that contains not less than 46.5% of ethoxyl groups is freely soluble in chloroform, ethanol (95%), ethyl acetate, methanol and toluene.

Specific ethylcellulose grades, or blends of different grades, may be used to obtain solutions of a desired viscosity. 5% (*w/v*) solutions of ethylcellulose in organic solvents show viscosities of 6~110mPa • s. The viscosity of solutions increases with an increase in the concentration of ethylcellulose. Solutions of higher viscosity tend to be composed of longer polymer chains and produce stronger and tougher films.

② *Stability and storage conditions*   Ethylcellulose is a stable and slightly hygroscopic material. The bulk material should be stored in a dry place and in a well-closed container at a temperature between 7~32℃. Ethylcellulose is chemically resistant to alkalis and to salt solutions and it is more sensitive to acidic materials than cellulose esters. Ethylcellulose is subject to oxidative degradation in the presence of sunlight or UV light at elevated temperatures, which may be prevented by the use of an antioxidant and a compound with light absorption properties between 230~340nm.

③ *Safety*   Ethylcellulose is generally regarded as a nontoxic, nonallergenic and nonirritant material. It is not metabolized following oral consumption, thus be widely used in oral and topical pharmaceutical formulations. But ethylcellulose is not recommended for use in parenteral products, which may be harmful to the kidneys.

(3) Applications in pharmaceutical formulation or technology   Ethylcellulose is widely used in oral and topical pharmaceutical formulations, as listed in Table 3-4.

Table 3-4. The usage of ethylcellulose in pharmaceutical formulations.

Usage	Concentration /%
Microencapsulation	10.0~20.0
Sustained release tablet coating	3.0~10.0
Tablet coating	1.0~3.0
Tablet granulation	1.0~3.0

The main use of ethylcellulose in oral formulations is as a hydrophobic coating agent for tablets and granules, in order to modify the release of a drug, to mask an unpleasant taste, or to improve the stability of a formulation. Usually, ethylcellulose is dissolved in an organic solvent or solvent mixture to produce water-insoluble ethylcellulose films. Higher viscosity grades of ethylcellulose tend to produce stronger and tougher films. The solubility of ethylcellulose films may be modified by the addition of hydroxypropyl-methylcellulose or a plasticizer in the solution. Ethylcellulose is compatible with numerous plasticizers, like diethyl phthalate, benzyl benzoate, refined mineral oils, stearic acid, stearyl alcohol, corn oil and so on. On the other hand, an aqueous polymer dispersion of ethylcellulose may also be used to produce ethylcellulose films and coat granules, where drug release is via diffusion through coats of hydrated ethylcellulose.

Ethylcellulose with high viscosity grades is usually used in drug microencapsulation. Release of a drug from an ethylcellulose microcapsule is a function of the microcapsule wall thickness.

In tablet formulations, ethylcellulose may also be used as a matrix former to modify drug release behavior. Ethylcellulose may additionally be employed as a binder by being blended dry or wet-granulated with a solvent such as ethanol (95%). It usually produces hard tablets with low friability and poor dissolution.

In topical formulations, ethylcellulose is used as a thickening agent in creams, lotions or gels.

3.2.5 Hydroxyethyl cellulose

(1) Polymer description　*Structural formula of hydroxyethyl cellulose*:

n, R=HOCH$_2$CH$_2$—, H

Hydroxyethyl cellulose (HEC) is a partially substituted poly(hydroxyethyl) ether of cellulose. It is available in several grades, varying in viscosity and degree of substitution.

Hydroxyethyl cellulose is usually prepared through a two-step procedure. Firstly, the purified cellulose is reacted with sodium hydroxide to produce swollen alkali cellulose which is chemically more reactive than untreated cellulose. The alkali cellulose is then reacted with ethylene oxide to produce a series of hydroxyethyl cellulose ethers. Though each anhydroglucose unit of the cellulose molecule has three hydroxyl groups and the maximum value of DS is 3, ethylene oxide can further react with additional hydroxyethyl groups in an end-to-end formation in this reaction. For hydroxyethyl cellulose, the manner of ethylene oxide added to cellulose is usually described by the molar substitution here. Molar substitution is defined as the average number or ethylene oxide molecules that have reacted with each anhydroglucose unit. Hence, theoretically there is no limit for molar substitution.

(2) Typical properties Hydroxyethyl cellulose occurs as a light tan or cream to white-colored, odorless and tasteless powder. It softens at 135~140℃ and decomposes at about 205℃.

Hydroxyethyl cellulose is hygroscopic. The amount of absorbed water depends upon the initial moisture content and the relative humidity of the surrounding air. Commercially available grades of hydroxyethyl cellulose contain less than 5% (w/w) of water.

① *Solubility* Hydroxyethyl cellulose is soluble in either hot or cold water, forming clear, smooth and uniform solutions. It is practically insoluble in acetone, ethanol, ether, toluene and most other organic solvents. However, hydroxyethyl cellulose can swell or be partially soluble in some polar organic solvents, such as the glycols.

The aqueous solution of hydroxyethyl cellulose is available in a wide range of viscosity from 2mPa • s to 20000mPa • s for a 2% (w/v) aqueous solution, which differs principally depending on the hydroxyethyl cellulose grades. Take NATROSOL® 250 Pharm HEC as an example, which is produced in Zwijndrecht (Netherlands) with the DS of 2.5, its viscosity varies regarding different grades, as shown in Table 3-5.

Table 3-5. NATROSOL 250 Pharm HEC is available in the following viscosity types.

Type	Typical 2% viscosity at $10s^{-1}$ and 20℃
NATROSOL 250 HHX Pharm	15000mPa • s
NATROSOL 250 HX Pharm	9000mPa • s
NATROSOL 250 M Pharm	5000mPa • s
NATROSOL 250 G Pharm	400mPa • s

② *Stability and storage conditions* Hydroxyethyl cellulose powder is a stable and hygroscopic material. Aqueous solutions of hydroxyethyl cellulose are relatively stable at pH=2~12 with the viscosity of solutions being largely unaffected. However, solutions are less stable below pH 5 due to hydrolysis. At high pH, oxidation may occur. Increasing temperature reduces the viscosity of aqueous hydroxyethyl cellulose solutions. Hydroxyethyl cellulose is subject to enzymatic degradation, so an antimicrobial preservative should be added to aqueous solutions for prolonged storage. Aqueous solutions of hydroxyethyl cellulose may also be sterilized by autoclaving.

③ *Incompatibilities* Hydroxyethyl cellulose is incompatible with zein and partially compatible with gelatin, methylcellulose, polyvinyl alcohol and starch. Hydroxyethyl cellulose has good tolerance for dissolved electrolytes while it may be salted out of solution when mixed with certain salt solutions like sodium carbonate 50% and saturated solutions of aluminum sulfate, sodium sulfate, sodium thiosulfate and zinc sulfate. Hydroxyethyl cellulose is also incompatible with certain fluorescent dyes or optical brighteners. Hydroxyethyl cellulose can be used with a wide variety of water-soluble antimicrobial preservatives except sodium pentachlorophenate, which would lead to an immediate viscosity increase of hydroxyethyl cellulose solutions.

③ *Safety* Hydroxyethyl cellulose is generally regarded as an essentially nontoxic and nonirritant material. Acute and subacute oral toxicity studies show that hydroxyethyl cellulose can be neither absorbed nor hydrolyzed in the rat gastrointestinal tract. It is used in oral pharmaceutical formulations, but is not recommended for use in parenteral products.

(3) Applications in pharmaceutical formulation or technology Hydroxyethyl cellulose is a nonionic and water soluble natural polymer widely used in pharmaceutical formulations. Hydroxyethyl cellulose is primarily used as a thickening agent in ophthalmic and topical formulations and it is also used as a binder or a film-coating agent for tablets.

3.2.6 Hydroxypropyl cellulose

(1) Polymer description *Structural formula of hydroxypropyl cellulose*:

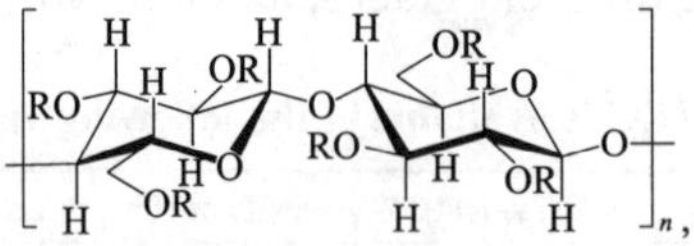

Hydroxypropyl cellulose is a partially substituted poly(hydroxypropyl) ether of cellulose. The content of hydroxypropoxy groups is in range of 53.4%~77.8% described by USPNF and BP. However, hydroxypropyl cellulose described in Chinese Pharmacopoeia refers to a low-substituted hydroxypropyl cellulose containing 5%~16% of hydroxypropoxy groups.

Commercially, hydroxypropyl cellulose is available in a number of different grades with different solution viscosities, and its molecular weight ranges between 50000 and 1250000.

The preparation of hydroxypropyl cellulose is similar as hydroxyethyl cellulose. The purified cellulose is reacted with sodium hydroxide to produce swollen alkali cellulose, which is then reacted with propylene oxide at elevated temperature and pressure. The propylene oxide can be substituted on the cellulose through an ether linkage at the three reactive hydroxyls present on each anhydroglucose monomer unit of the cellulose chain. The secondary hydroxyl present in the substituent hydroxypropyl groups is available for further reaction with the propylene oxide. This results in the formation of side chains containing more than one mole of combined propylene oxide in hydroxyethyl cellulose.

(2) Typical properties　Hydroxypropyl cellulose is a white to slightly yellow-colored, odorless and tasteless powder. It is a thermoplastic polymer, which softens at 130℃ and chars at 260~275℃. Hydroxypropyl cellulose is hygroscopic. The typical equilibrium moisture content values at 25℃ are 4% w/w at 50% relative humidity and 12% w/w at 84% relative humidity.

① *Solubility*　Hydroxypropyl cellulose is freely soluble in water below 38℃ forming a smooth, clear and colloidal solution. But it is insoluble in hot water and is precipitated as a highly swollen floc at a temperature between 40~45℃.

Hydroxypropyl cellulose is soluble in many polar organic solvents such as dimethyl formamide, dimethyl sulfoxide, dioxane, ethanol, methanol, propan-2-ol (95%) and propylene glycol. Although the higher viscosity grades of hydroxypropyl cellulose show weak solubility, their solution quality in borderline solvents can often be greatly improved by the use of small quantities (5%~15%) of a co-solvent. For example, solutions of *Klucel*® *HF*❶ (Molecular weight≈1150000) in dichloromethane have a granular texture, while a smooth solution may be produced by adding 10% methanol.

② *Stability and storage conditions*　Hydroxypropyl cellulose powder is a stable material, which should be stored in a well-closed container in a cool and dry place.

Aqueous solutions of hydroxypropyl cellulose have optimum stability at pH=6.0~8.0. However, a decrease in solution viscosity occurs at low pH due to acid hydrolysis and at high pH due to alkali-catalyzed oxidation degradation. Ultraviolet light and certain enzymes, produced by microbial action, will also degrade hydroxypropyl cellulose. For prolonged storage, aqueous hydroxypropyl cellulose solutions should therefore be protected from light and heat with an antimicrobial preservative added.

③ *Incompatibilities*　Hydroxypropyl cellulose in solution is compatible with a number of high molecular weight, high boiling waxes and oils. It demonstrates some incompatibility with substituted phenol derivatives, such as methylparaben and

---

❶ *Klucel*® hydroxypropylcellulose (HPC) is a nonionic water-soluble cellulose ether with a versatile combination of properties. Aqualon holds a Drug Master File on Klucel hydroxypropylcellulose.

propylparaben. The presence of anionic polymers may increase the viscosity of hydroxypropyl cellulose solutions. In addition, hydroxypropyl cellulose may be salted out in the presence of high concentrations of other dissolved materials like inorganic salts, since the dissolved materials will compete water hydrated with polymer and influence the balance of the hydrophilic-lipophilic properties of the polymers.

④ *Safety*　Hydroxypropylcellulose is generally regarded as an essentially nontoxic and nonirritant material, which is included in the FDA Inactive Ingredients Guide for oral capsules and tablets and transdermal preparations. Adverse reactions to hydroxypropyl cellulose are rare. There have been few reports on hypersensitivity and edema of the eyelids associated with hydroxypropyl cellulose as a solid ocular insert. A single case of allergic contact dermatitis was reported for hydroxypropyl cellulose used in a transdermal estradiol patch. Excessive consumption of hydroxypropyl cellulose may however have a laxative effect.

(3) Applications in pharmaceutical formulation or technology　Hydroxypropyl cellulose is widely used in oral and topical pharmaceutical formulations.

In oral products, hydroxypropyl cellulose is primarily used in tableting as a binder [2%~6% (w/w) in either wet or dry granulation or direct compression tableting processes], film-coating [5% (w/w) of either aqueous or ethanolic solutions] and extended release matrix former [15%~35% (w/w)]. The release rate of a drug increases with decreasing viscosity of hydroxypropyl cellulose. The addition of an anionic surfactant may increase the hydroxypropyl cellulose viscosity and hence decrease the release rate of a drug. Hydroxypropyl cellulose is also used in microencapsulation processes as a thickening agent.

In topical formulations, hydroxypropyl cellulose is used in transdermal patches and ophthalmic preparations.

It is noted that the low-substituted hydroxypropyl cellulose is insoluble in water but swells. It can be used as a tablet disintegrant or as a sustained release tablet matrix.

3.2.7　Hydroxypropyl methylcellulose

(1) Polymer description　*Structural formula of hydroxypropyl methylcellulose*:

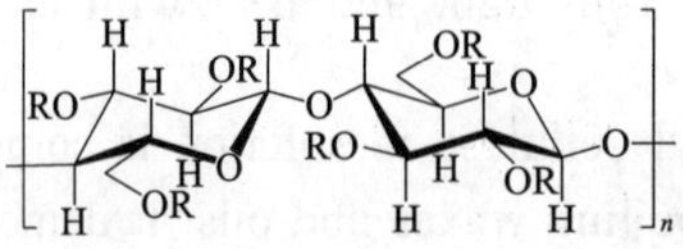

Hydroxypropyl methylcellulose (HPMC) is a partly O-methylated and O-(2-hydroxypropylated) cellulose. It is available in several grades with different viscosity and substitution. Hydroxypropyl methylcellulose defined in the USP XXII specifies the substitution type by appending a four digit number to the nonproprietary name, e.g. hydroxypropyl methylcellulose 1828. The first two digits refer to the approximate percentage content of the methoxy group (OCH_3). The second two digits refer to the approximate percentage content of the hydroxy-propoxy group ($OCH_2CHOHCH_3$). Four grades of hydroxypropyl methylcellulose are included in USP as shown in Table 3-6. Molecular weight is approximately 10000~1500000.

Table 3-6. Four grades of hydroxypropyl methylcellulose included in USP.

HPMC grads	$-OCH_3$ /%	$OCH_2CHOHCH_3$ /%
1828	16.5 ~ 20.0	23.0 ~ 32.0
2208	19.0 ~ 24.0	4.0 ~ 12.0
2906	27.0 ~ 30.0	4.0 ~ 7.5
2910	28.0 ~ 30.0	7.0 ~ 12.0

The preparation of hydroxypropyl methylcellulose is similar with hydroxypropyl cellulose as mentioned before. A swollen alkali cellulose is obtained from purified form of cellulose following the reaction with chloromethane and propylene oxide, which will produce methylhydroxypropyl ethers of cellulose. The fibrous reaction product is purified and ground to a fine and uniform powder or granules.

(2) Typical properties　Hydroxypropyl methylcellulose is an odorless and tasteless, white or creamy-white colored fibrous or granular powder. It chars at 225~230℃ and the glass transition temperature is 170~180℃.

① *Solubility*　Hydroxypropyl methylcellulose is soluble in cold water, forming a viscous colloidal solution. To prepare an aqueous solution, it is recommended that hydroxypropyl methylcellulose is dispersed and thoroughly hydrated in about 20%~30% of the required amount of hot water (80~90℃). Cold water is then be added to produce the required volume. Additionally, hydroxypropyl methylcellulose undergoes a reversible sol to gel transformation upon heating and cooling respectively. The gel point is about 50~90℃, depending upon the grade of material.

Hydroxypropyl methylcellulose is practically insoluble in chloroform, ethanol (95%) and ether, but soluble in mixtures of ethanol and dichloromethane, and mixtures of methanol and dichloromethane. Solutions prepared using organic solvents tend to be more viscous.

② *Stability and storage conditions*　Hydroxypropyl methylcellulose powder is a stable material with some hygroscopicity. It should be stored in a well-closed container in a cool and dry place.

Hydroxypropyl methylcellulose solutions are stable at pH=3~11, providing good viscosity stability during long-term storage. Increasing temperature reduces the viscosity of solutions, and the coagulated polymer must be redispersed on cooling by shaking. However, aqueous solutions are liable to microbial spoilage and should be preserved with an antimicrobial preservative. Aqueous solutions may be sterilized by autoclaving.

③ *Safety* Hydroxypropyl methylcellulose is generally regarded as a nontoxic and nonirritant material although excessive oral consumption may have a laxative effect. The WHO has not specified an acceptable daily intake for hydroxypropyl methylcellulose since the levels consumed are not considered to represent a hazard to health.

(3) Applications in pharmaceutical formulation or technology Hydroxypropyl methylcellulose is widely used in oral and topical pharmaceutical formulations.

In oral products, hydroxypropyl methylcellulose is primarily used as a tablet binder, in film coating and as an extended release tablet matrix. Concentrations of 2%~5% (w/w) may be used as a binder in either wet or dry granulation processes. High viscosity grades may be used to retard the release of water-soluble drugs from a matrix. Concentrations of 2%~10% (w/w) are used as film-forming solutions to film-coat tablets. Lower viscosity grades are used in aqueous film-coating solutions while higher viscosity grades are used with organic solvents.

For example, a hydrophilic HPMC matrix tablet containing melatonin (MT) was prepared by direct compression and was formulated as a function of HPMC viscosity grades. The poorly water-soluble MT was released from the HPMC matrices by the diffusion of the gelatinous layer, followed by the erosion of the gel regardless of the testing pH. As the viscosity of the HPMC polymer increased, the release rate had a tendency to decrease (Figure 3-5)[5].

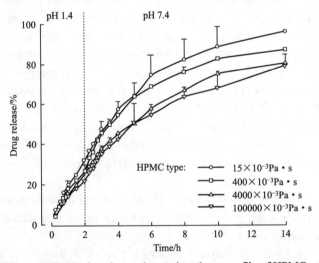

Figure 3-5. Effect of HPMC viscosity grades on the release profile of HPMC matrix tablets.

Hydroxypropyl methylcellulose is also used as a suspending and thickening agent in topical formulations, particularly in ophthalmic preparations. Concentrations of

0.45%~1.0% (*w/w*) may be added as a thickening agent to vehicles for eye-drops and artificial tear solutions. Compared with methylcellulose, hydroxypropyl methylcellulose solutions have greater clarity and are therefore preferred in formulations for ophthalmic use.

In addition, hydroxypropyl methylcellulose is used as an emulsifier, suspending agent and stabilizing agent in topical gels and ointments. As a protective colloid, it can prevent droplets and particles from coalescing or agglomerating, thus inhibiting the formation of sediments. Hydroxypropyl methylcellulose is also used as a wetting agent for hard contact lenses.

3.2.8 Carboxymethylcellulose sodium

(1) Polymer description *Structural formula of carboxymethylcellulose sodium*:

n, R=CH$_2$COONa

Carboxymethylcellulose sodium is the sodium salt of a polycarboxymethyl ether of cellulose, with the typical molecular weight in 90000~700000 and the degree of substitution in 0.7~1.2. A number of grades of carboxymethylcellulose sodium are commercially available, and the most frequently used grade has a degree of substitution (DS) of 0.7.

The preparation procedure is as below: Alkali cellulose is firstly obtained by steeping cellulose obtained from wood pulp or cotton fibers in sodium hydroxide solution. The alkali cellulose is then reacted with sodium monochloroacetate to produce carboxymethylcellulose sodium. Sodium chloride and sodium glycolate are obtained as by-products of this etherification.

(2) Typical properties   Carboxymethylcellulose sodium occurs as a white to almost white, odorless and granular powder. Carboxymethylcellulose sodium is hygroscopic. Under high humidity conditions it can absorb a large quantity (> 50%) of water.

① *Solubility*   Carboxymethylcellulose sodium is practically insoluble in acetone, ethanol, ether and toluene. It is easily dispersed in water at all temperatures, forming clear and colloidal solutions. The aqueous solubility varies with the degree of substitution.

Various grades of carboxymethylcellulose sodium are commercially available showing different viscosities. Aqueous 1% (*w/v*) solutions of carboxymethylcellulose exhibit viscosities in range of 5~4000mPa • s. An increase in concentration results in an increase in aqueous solution viscosity.

② *Stability and storage conditions*　Carboxymethylcellulose sodium is stable but hygroscopic. In tablets, this has been associated with a decrease in tablet hardness and an increase in disintegration time. The bulk material should be stored in a well-closed container in a cool and dry place.

Aqueous solutions of carboxymethylcellulose sodium are stable at pH=2~10. Precipitation can occur below pH=2 while viscosity rapidly decreases above pH=10. Generally, solutions exhibit maximum viscosity and stability at pH=7~9. Aqueous solutions stored for prolonged periods should contain an antimicrobial preservative.

Carboxymethylcellulose sodium may be sterilized in the dry state by maintaining it at a temperature of 160℃ for 1 hour. However, this process results in a significant decrease in viscosity and some deterioration in the properties of solutions. Aqueous solutions may similarly be sterilized by heating although this also results in some reduction in viscosity. Sterilization of solutions by gamma irradiation also results in reduction in viscosity.

③ *Incompatibilities*　Carboxymethylcellulose sodium is incompatible with strongly acidic solutions and with the soluble salts of iron and some other metals, such as aluminum, mercury and zinc. It is also incompatible with xanthan gum. Precipitation occurs when carboxymethylcellulose sodium solutions are mixed with ethanol (95%). Carboxymethylcellulose sodium can form complexes with gelatin and collagen. It is additionally capable of precipitating certain positive charged proteins.

④ *Safety*　Carboxymethylcellulose sodium is generally regarded as a nontoxic and nonirritant material. However, oral consumption of large amounts of carboxymethylcellulose sodium can have a laxative effect (therapeutically 4~10g, in daily divided doses). In animal studies, subcutaneous administration of carboxymethylcellulose sodium has been found to cause inflammation and hypersensitive reaction.

(3) Applications in pharmaceutical formulation or technology　Carboxymethylcellulose sodium is widely used in oral and topical pharmaceutical formulations primarily for its viscosity-increasing properties. Viscous aqueous solutions of carboxymethylcellulose sodium are used to suspend powders intended for oral and parenteral administration. Higher concentrations (4%~6%) of the medium viscosity grade is used to produce gels which can be used as the base for pastes. Carboxymethylcellulose sodium is additionally one of the main ingredients of self adhesive ostomy, wound care and dermatological patches where it is used to absorb wound exudate or transepidermal water and sweat.

Carboxymethylcellulose sodium may also be used as a tablet binder and disintegrant, or be used to stabilize emulsions.

3.2.9　Carboxymethylcellulose calcium

(1) Polymer description　Carboxymethylcellulose calcium is the calcium salt of a

polycarboxymethyl ether of cellulose, which substituted degree is similar as carboxymethylcellulose sodium. Carboxymethylcellulose calcium is obtained by the conversion of carboxymethylcellulose sodium into the calcium salt.

(2) Typical properties   Carboxymethylcellulose calcium occurs as a white to yellowish-white colored and hygroscopic powder.

① *Solubility*   Carboxymethylcellulose calcium is insoluble in water, but swells to twice its volume to form a suspension. It is also practically insoluble in acetone, chloroform, ethanol (95%) and ether.

② *Safety*   Carboxymethylcellulose calcium is generally regarded as a nontoxic and nonirritant material, similarly as carboxymethylcellulose sodium.

(3) Applications in pharmaceutical formulation or technology   The main use of carboxymethylcellulose calcium is in tablet formulations as a binder, diluent and disintegrant. The maximum concentration used in tablet formulations is up to 15% (*w/w*), while above this concentration tablet hardness is reduced. Although carboxymethylcellulose calcium is insoluble in water, it is an effective tablet disintegrant since it swells to several times its original bulk while in contact with water.

Carboxymethylcellulose calcium is also used as a suspending or viscosity increasing agent in oral and topical pharmaceutical formulations, just as carboxymethylcellulose sodium functions.

3.2.10   Cellulose acetate phthalate

(1) Polymer description   *Structural formula of cellulose acetate phthalate*:

Cellulose acetate phthalate is a kind of cellulose derivate in which about half the hydroxyl groups are acetylated and about a quarter are esterified with one of the two acid groups from phthalic acid. It is noted that the other acid group belonging to phthalic acid is free in cellulose acetate phthalate.

Cellulose acetate phthalate is produced by the reaction of the partial acetate ester of cellulose with phthalic anhydride in the presence of a tertiary organic base, such as pyridine.

(2) Typical properties   Cellulose acetate phthalate occurs as white and free-flowing powder or colorless flakes. It is tasteless and odorless or may have a slight odor of acetic acid. Cellulose acetate phthalate is hygroscopic, so precautions are necessary to avoid moisture. Melting point of cellulose acetate phthalate is 192℃. Glass transition temperature is 160~170℃.

① *Solubility* Cellulose acetate phthalate is soluble in certain buffered aqueous solutions at pH>6. It is also soluble in cyclic ethers, esters, ether alcohols, ketones and certain solvent mixtures like acetone/ethanol (1:1). When using mixed solvents, it is important to dissolve the cellulose acetate phthalate in the solvent with the greater dissolving power, and then to add the second solvent. Cellulose acetate phthalate should always be added to the solvent instead of the reverse. Cellulose acetate phthalate is practically insoluble in water, alcohols, hydrocarbons and chlorinated hydrocarbons.

② *Stability and storage conditions* Cellulose acetate phthalate is stable if stored in a well-closed container in a cool and dry place. It hydrolyzes slowly under prolonged adverse conditions, such as high temperature and humidity, which results in an increase in free acid content, viscosity and odor of acetic acid.

③ *Safety* Cellulose acetate phthalate is generally regarded as a nontoxic material in oral pharmaceutical products, which is included in the FDA Inactive Ingredients Guide (oral capsules and tablets). Cellulose acetate phthalate is also included in nonparenteral medicines licensed in the UK.

(3) Applications in pharmaceutical formulation or technology Cellulose acetate phthalate is commonly applied to solid dosage forms as an enteric film coating material, or as a matrix binder for tablets and capsules by direct compression. It is noted that the free carboxylic acid group of phthalic acid moiety remains unesterified, leading to incompatibility of cellulose acetate phthalate with acid sensitive drugs.

The coating of cellulose acetate ph can be put into practice from organic or aqueous solvent systems. A 15% (*w/w*) solution in acetone with a moisture content of 0.4% is a good coating solution with a honey-like consistency and viscosity at 50~90mPa • s. Such coatings resist prolonged contact with the strongly acidic gastric fluid, but soften and swell in the mildly acidic or neutral intestinal environment. The addition of plasticizers improves the water resistance of this coating material. Cellulose acetate phthalate films are permeable to certain ionic substances, such as potassium iodide and ammonium chloride. In such cases, an appropriate sealer subcoat should be used. It may also be used in combination with other coating agents to control drug release, e.g. ethylcellulose.

◆ 本节中文导读 ◆

纤维素是自然界中分布最广、含量最多的一种多糖，是组成植物细胞壁的主要成分。纤维素的结构为长链线型高分子化合物，由 D-吡喃型葡萄糖单元（失水葡萄糖）通过 β-1,4 糖苷键连接而成。纤维素大分子的每个葡萄糖单元中有 3 个羟基，其中 2 个为仲羟基，另一个为伯羟基，纤维素的氧化、酯化、醚化、分子间形成氢键、吸水、溶胀以及接枝共聚等都与纤维素分子中存在大量羟基有关。由于纤维素分子量大，纤维素分子大量羟基之间形成的分子间和分子内氢键作用非常之大，形成结晶区。纤维素是由很多微晶区和非晶区交织在一起形成的多晶。因此，纤维素虽然具有吸湿性，但不溶于水和常用有机溶剂。纤维素在碱液中发生溶胀。纤维素衍生物辅料产品包括纤维素酯、纤维素醚和纤维素醚酯，它们的性质与纤维素有明显差异，受到如下因素的影响，包括：取代基团的结构和性质、取代基的数量、取代基在纤维素衍生物分子中分布的均匀性、分子量及其分布。

（1）微晶纤维素（microcrystalline cellulose） 微晶纤维素是一种部分解聚的纤维素，从植物纤维素部分水解而制得，为白色、无臭、无味、由多孔微粒组成的晶体粉末。微晶纤维素微溶于 5%氢氧化钠溶液，不溶于水、稀酸和多数有机溶剂；有吸湿性，性质稳定。微晶纤维素广泛应用在口服药物制剂和食品中，是相对无毒和无刺激性的物质。用于药物制剂，主要是在口服片剂和胶囊剂中作为胶黏剂或稀释剂，可用于湿法制粒和直接压片。除此以外，微晶纤维素还有一定的润湿和崩解性。

（2）粉状纤维素（powdered cellulose） 粉状纤维素为粒径大小不一的粉末，将从纤维性植物中获得的α-纤维素浆状物通过纯化及机械法降低粒径而制得。粉状纤维素可分散于大部分液体中，在水/稀酸和大部分有机溶剂中几乎不溶，在5%(质量浓度) 的氢氧化钠溶液中微溶。粉状纤维素是稳定的稍有吸湿性的物质，流动性不好，但有好的压实性。低结晶度的粉状纤维素可作为直接压片用辅料。粉状纤维素可用作片剂稀释剂和硬胶囊的填充剂；用作散剂辅料；用作口服水性混悬液的助悬剂。在栓剂制备中，粉状纤维素用来降低药物沉降作用。

（3）甲基纤维素（methylcellulose） 甲基纤维素中约 27%～32%的羟基被甲氧基取代，不同级别的甲基纤维素具有不同的聚合度，其分子量范围在 10000～220000 之间。甲基纤维素在丙酮、甲醇、氯仿、乙醇、乙醚、甲苯、饱和盐溶液和热水中几乎不溶，溶于冰醋酸及等量混合的乙醇和氯仿溶液中。有良好的亲水性，在冷水中膨胀生成澄明及乳白色的黏稠胶体溶液。甲基纤维素广泛应用于口服制剂和局部用制剂中：口服液体制剂的助悬剂或增稠剂，局部用制剂产品如乳膏和凝胶的增稠剂，可延迟混悬液的沉降并增加药物在胃肠道的接触时间；片剂中的胶黏剂和崩解剂，片心的包衣，包糖衣前包于片心外作隔离层。

（4）乙基纤维素（ethylcellulose, EC） 乙基纤维素是纤维素的乙基醚。乙基纤维素基本不吸湿，不溶于甘油和水。乙氧基含量低于 46.5%的乙基纤维素易溶于氯仿、乙酸甲酯、四氢呋喃及芳香烃与 95%乙醇的混合物。而乙氧基含量高于46.5%的乙基纤维素易溶于氯仿、95%乙醇、乙酸乙酯、甲醇及甲苯。乙基纤维素稳定，耐碱（稀碱或浓碱）耐盐，广泛应用于口服和外用制剂中：如片剂和颗粒的疏水性包衣材料，片剂的胶黏剂，缓释片的骨架材料，软膏、洗剂或凝胶中的增稠剂。高黏度乙基纤维素可用于药物微囊化。但用乙基纤维素制得的片子硬、脆性低、溶出度差。

（5）羟乙基纤维素（hydroxyethyl cellulose, HEC） 羟乙基纤维素为纤维素的羟乙基醚，由于醚化反应后的羟乙基上也含有羟基，可进一步与环氧乙烷反应，对应纤维素脱水葡萄糖单元的一个羟基上可能存在不止一分子的环氧乙烷单元。羟乙基纤维素可溶于热水和冷水中，形成透明、均匀的溶液。在丙酮、乙醇、醚、甲苯及其他多数有机溶剂中几乎不溶。加热羟乙基纤维素水溶液，不形成凝胶，这是羟乙基纤维素与羟丙纤维素和羟丙甲纤维素的不同之处。羟乙基纤维素主要用作眼科制剂和局部用药制剂的增稠剂，也可用作片剂的胶黏剂和膜包衣材料，在干眼症、隐形眼镜的润滑剂中都含有羟乙基纤维素。

（6）羟丙纤维素（hydroxypropyl cellulose, HPC） 羟丙纤维素为纤维素的聚羟丙基醚。市售的羟丙纤维素有不同规格，其水溶液有不同黏度，分子量范围为 50000～1250000。羟丙纤维素在烷烃、芳烃、四氯化碳、石油馏出物、甘油以及油类中几乎不溶，在许多冷的或热的极性有机溶剂中溶解，如二甲酰胺、二甲亚砜、乙醇、甲醇、丙二醇。羟丙纤维素与低于 38℃的水可混溶形成透明的胶体溶液。在热水中不溶，在 40～45℃形成高度溶胀的絮状沉淀。羟丙纤维素广泛应用于各种口服和局部用制剂中，在纳米囊化学工艺过程中作为增稠剂，也在透皮贴剂或眼科制剂中使用。

（7）羟丙甲纤维素（hydroxypropyl methylcellulose，HPMC） 羟丙甲纤维素为部分 O-甲基化，部分 O-(2-羟丙基化) 纤维素。市售品有不同黏度、不同取代度的各种级别产品，分子量大约为 10000～1500000。羟丙甲纤维素在氯仿、乙醇（95%）和乙醚中几乎不溶，在乙醇和二氯甲烷混合液、甲醇和二氯甲烷混合液、以及水和乙醇混合液中溶解。羟丙甲纤维素可用作片剂的胶黏剂，片剂和胶囊剂骨架的阻滞剂，片剂薄膜包衣，眼科制剂的助悬剂和增稠剂，局部用凝胶剂和软膏剂的乳化剂、混悬剂和稳定剂。羟丙甲纤维素也可作隐形眼镜的湿润剂。

（8）羧甲基纤维素钠（carboxymethylcellulose sodium, CMCNa） 羧甲基纤维素钠为纤维素的羧甲基醚钠盐，分子量为 90000～700000。羧甲纤维素钠几乎不溶于丙酮、乙醇、乙醚和甲苯，在水中易分散，形成透明、胶状溶液。羧甲纤维素钠由于其增黏特性被广泛用于口服和局部用药物制剂。它的黏性水溶液在局部、口服或注射用制剂中用作助悬剂，在片剂中用作胶黏剂和崩解剂，还可用于稳定乳剂。羧甲纤维素钠还是自黏合造漏术、伤口护理材料和皮肤用贴剂中的主要成分之一，可吸收伤口的分泌物或皮肤的汗水。交联羧甲基纤维素钠由于分子为交联结构，不溶于水，具有良好吸水溶胀性，有助于片剂中药物溶出和崩解，是一种超级崩解剂。

（9）羧甲基纤维素钙（carboxymethylcellulose calcium, CMCCa） 羧甲基纤维素钙为纤维素羧甲基醚的钙盐，从木浆或棉纤维中得到的纤维素经羧甲基化后转化成钙盐。羧甲基纤维素钙几乎不溶于丙酮、氯仿、乙醇（95%）和乙醚，不溶于水，但吸水溶胀到原体积两倍形成混悬液。羧甲纤维素钙具有黏结力适中、表观密度高、稳定性好、无毒副作用等特点，可作为助悬剂、增稠剂、丸剂和片剂的崩解剂、胶黏剂和分散剂，所制药片硬度高、口感好。

（10）醋酸纤维素酞酸酯（cellulose acetate phthalate） 醋酸纤维素酞酸酯又称纤维醋法酯。PhEur2002 和 USPNF20 中将纤维醋法酯描述为含有 21.5%～26.0% 的乙酰基和 30.0%～26.0%的邻苯二甲酸基的部分乙酰化纤维素衍生物，其结构特点是具有游离的羧基。纤维醋法酯有吸湿性，在水、乙醇、氯代烷和烷烃中几乎不溶，在酮、酯和某些混合溶剂中可溶。纤维醋法酯广泛应用于口服制剂中，如肠溶包衣材料，或是片剂和胶囊剂的骨架胶黏剂。纤维醋法酯的包衣层可以耐受长时间与强酸性胃液的接触，但在弱碱性或中性的肠液环境中可以溶解。纤维醋法酯可与其他包衣剂如乙基纤维素合用，用于控释给药制剂。

3.3 Other natural polymers in pharmaceutics

3.3.1 Chitin/chitosan

(1) Polymer description   Chitin is the second most abundant polysaccharide in nature, next to cellulose, which exists in the exoskeleton of crustacean, insects, and some fungi. The main commercial sources of chitin are the shell wastes of shrimp, lobster, krill and crab. Several million tons of chitin are harvested annually in the world. Structurally, chitin is poly-(N-acetyl-2-amino-2-deoxy-D-glucopyranose), a structure very similar to that of cellulose, except that the acetyl amino group replaces the hydroxyl group on the C-2 position.

Chitosan {poly [β(1→4) 2-amino-2-deoxy-β-D-glucan]} is a linear polyaminosaccharide obtained by the N-deacetylation of chitin. It is difficult to carry out complete N-deacetylation of chitin. Thus, the chitosan molecule is a copolymer of N-acetylglucosamine and glucosamine. The degree of deacetylation (%DD) in commercial chitosans ranges from 60% to 100%, which can be determined by NMR spectroscopy. And the molecular weight of commercially produced chitosan is between 3800 and 20000. Generally, chitosan has a rigid crystalline structure through inter- and intramolecular hydrogen bonding.

Structural formula of chitin and chitosan:

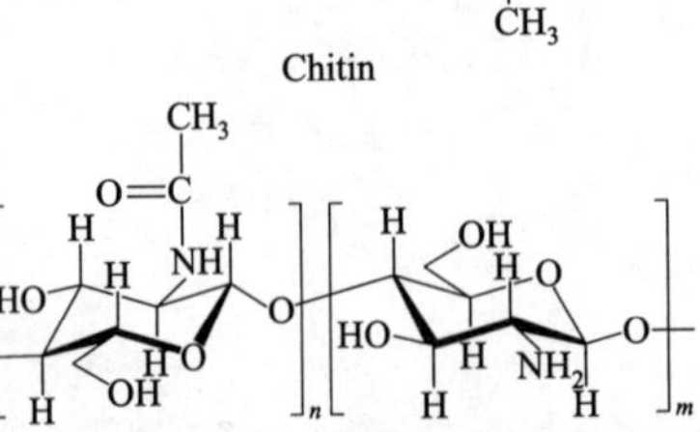

Chitin

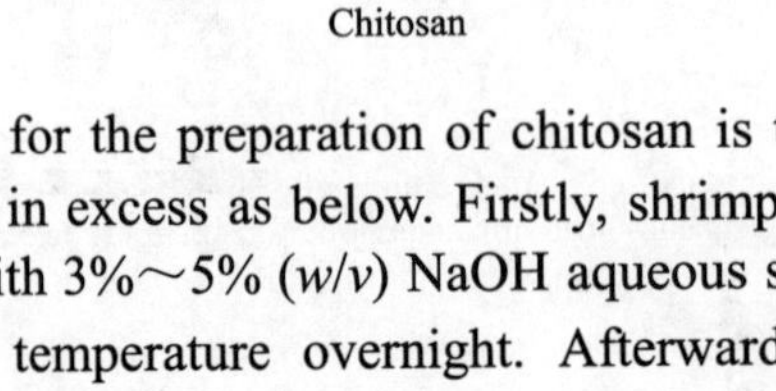

Chitosan

A common method for the preparation of chitosan is the deacetylation of chitin using sodium hydroxide in excess as below. Firstly, shrimp or crab shell proteins are removed by treatment with 3%~5% (w/v) NaOH aqueous solution at 80~90℃ for a few hours or at room temperature overnight. Afterward, the product's inorganic constituents are removed by treatment with 3%~5% (*w/v*) HCl aqueous solution at room temperature giving a white to beige colored sample of chitin. Then, chitin samples are treated with an aqueous 40%~45% (*w/v*) NaOH solution at 90~120℃ for 4~5 h, resulting in N-deacetylation of chitin. The insoluble precipitate is washed with water to give a crude sample of chitosan. The crude sample is dissolved in aqueous 2% (*w/v*) acetic acid. The insoluble material is removed giving a clear supernatant solution which is neutralized with NaOH solution, resulting in a purified sample of chitosan as a white precipitate. Further purification may be necessary to prepare medical and pharmaceutical grade chitosan.

The conditions used for deacetylation will determine the polymer molecular weight and the degree of deacetylation. This reaction pathway, when allowed to go to completion (complete deacetylation) yields up to 98% product.

(2) Typical properties　Chitin is translucent, pliable, resilient and quite tough in its unmodified form. As mentioned previously, chitin may be structurally described as cellulose with one hydroxyl group on each monomer replaced with an acetyl amine group. This allows for increased hydrogen bonding between adjacent polymers, giving the chitin-polymer matrix increased strength. Chitin is insoluble in water and most organic solvents, except for some acids such as trifluoroacetic acid.

Chitosan is a weak base with a pKa value of D-glucosamine about at 6.5. Therefore, it is insoluble at neutral and alkaline pH values. In acidic medium, the amine groups in chitosan are protonated resulting in a soluble and positively charged polysaccharide. That means chitosan is soluble by making salts with inorganic and organic acids such as hydrochloric acid, acetic acid, glutamic acid and lactic acid, where chitosan has a charge density dependent on pH and the DD-value (%). The positive charge makes chitosan bioadhesive which readily binds to negatively charged surfaces such as mucosal membranes. And chitosan can form gels by interacting with many multivalent anions.

In addition, the viscosity of chitosan solution is affected by factors such as degree of deacetylation, concentration and temperature. Increasing degree of deacetylation increases the viscosity, which can be explained by the fact that high and low deacetylated chitosan have different conformations. Chitosan molecule has a rodlike shape or a coiled shape at low degree of deacetylation due to the low charge density in polymer chain, while it shows an extended conformation with a more flexible chain when it is highly deacetylated because of the charge repulsion in the molecule. Also, the viscosity increases as the chitosan concentration increases and the temperature decreases.

Chitosan is biocompatible and biodegradable. Toxicity of chitosan depends on different factors such as degree of deacetylation, molecular weight, purity, and route of administration. Chitosan has low oral toxicity with an LD_{50} in rats of 16g/kg. Though it is not approved by FDA for drug delivery, purified quantities of chitosans are available for biomedical applications.

The pharmaceutical requirements of chitosan are as follows: particle size <30μm, density between 1.35g/cc and 1.40g/cc, pH=6.5～7.5, insoluble in water, and partially soluble in acids.

(3) Applications in pharmaceutical formulation or technology　Chitin's properties as a flexible and strong material make it favorable as surgical thread. Chitin has been reported to have some unusual properties that accelerate healing of wounds in humans.

As for chitosan, it is more attractive for the development of conventional and novel pharmaceutical products due to the unique physical and chemical properties such as the cationic charge in acidic medium [6]. Chitosan can be added in the preparation of tablet dosage forms. When chitosan was used as a binder in wet granulation, the binding efficiency was less than that of hydroxypropyl methylcellulose, but more than that of methylcellulose or sodium carboxymethyl cellulose. When chitosan was used in tablets at a concentration above 5% (w/w), its disintegration efficiency was higher than starch and microcrystalline cellulose.

There have been various examples of chitosan microspheres used for drug delivery. Chitosan microspheres can be prepared by different methods, such as crosslinking with glutaraldehyde, interfacial acylation, precipitation, spray-drying technique, ionotropic gelation, solvent evaporation and capillary extrusion. Chitosan can provide sustained release of drugs when used in oral drug formulations. Moreover, chitosan can be used as a bioadhesive polymer to increase residence time of dosage forms at mucosal sites, inhibit enzymes, and increase the permeability of protein and peptide drugs across mucosal membranes. A number of investigations have shown that chitosan could be used as a mucosal vaccine carrier and may have adjuvant effect.

Chitosan networks can serve as pH-sensitive swelling system for region-specific drug delivery in the gastrointestinal tract. Recently chitosan was reported to be degraded by the microflora available in the colon, resulting in the potential for colon-specific drug delivery.

Chitosan could also be used as a carrier of DNA for gene therapy. The cationically charged chitosan will form polyelectrolyte complexes with the negatively charged plasmid DNA, to inhibit degradation of DNA by DNase and to improve the bioavailability of the plasmid DNA delivered into the body. Though the transfection efficiency is limited, chitosan is promising in gene delivery system for its low toxicity. Moreover, chitosan could be easily modified by coupling with specific ligands, such as lactose, so the chitosan-DNA complex could be targeted to cells that express a galactose-binding membrane lectin[7].

3.3.2　Alginate and sodium/calcium alginate

(1) Polymer description　*Structural formula of alginic acid and sodium alginate*:

Alginic acid

Sodium alginate

Alginic acid, also called alginate, is an anionic polysaccharide distributed widely in the cell walls of brown seaweed. It is a linear copolymer consisting mainly of residues of (1-4)-linked β-D-mannuronate (M) and (1-4)-linked α-L-glucuronate (G). The monomers can appear in homopolymeric blocks of consecutive G-residues (G-blocks), consecutive M-residues (M-blocks) or alternating M and G-residues (MG-blocks). The molecular weight is typically 20000~200000.

Sodium alginate consists chiefly of the sodium salt of alginic acid. A number of different grades of sodium alginate, which have different solution viscosities, are commercially available. Many different alginate salts and derivatives are also commercially available including: ammonium alginate, calcium alginate, magnesium alginate and potassium alginate.

The manufacture of alginic acid and sodium alginate is described as below. The seaweed is harvested, crushed, and treated with dilute alkali to extract the alginic acid. The alginic acid is then neutralized with sodium bicarbonate to form sodium alginate.

(2) Typical properties   Alginic acid is a tasteless, practically odorless, white to yellowish-white colored and fibrous powder. Similarly, sodium alginate occurs as a tasteless and odorless, white to pale yellowish-brown colored powder.

① Solubility   Alginic acid is practically insoluble in ethanol (95%) and other organic solvents. It swells in water and is capable of absorbing 200~300 times its own weight in water. Alginic acid is soluble in alkali hydroxides, producing viscous solutions. Various grades of alginic acid are commercially available, varying in their molecular weight and viscosity. Alginic acid dispersions are best prepared by pouring the alginic acid slowly and steadily into vigorously stirred water. Dispersions should be stirred for approximately 30 minutes. At low concentrations, the viscosity of an alginic acid dispersion may be increased by the addition of a calcium salt, such as calcium citrate. Here, two G blocks of adjacent polymer chains can be cross-linked with multivalent cations (e.g., Ca^{2+}) through interactions with the carboxylic groups in the sugars, which lead to the formation of a gel network as shown in Figure 3-6. The overall gel stiffness depends on the polymer molecular weight distribution, the M/G ratio and the stoichiometry of the alginate with the chelating cation.

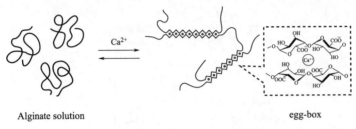

Alginate solution   egg-box

Figure 3-6. Schematic procedure of the gel formation by the interaction
between alginate and calcium ion.

Sodium alginate is practically insoluble in ethanol, ether and ethanol/water mixtures (where the ethanol content is greater than 30%). It is also practically insoluble in other organic solvents and acids (pH<3). Sodium alginate is slowly soluble in water, forming a viscous colloidal solution. Viscosity may vary depending upon concentration, pH, temperature or the presence of metal ions. The viscosity decreases above pH=10.

② *Stability and storage conditions*　Alginic acid hydrolyzes slowly at warm temperature producing a material with a lower molecular weight and lower dispersion viscosity. It should be stored in a well-closed container in a cool and dry place.

Sodium alginate is a hygroscopic material. The bulk material should be stored in an airtight container in a cool and dry place. Aqueous solutions of sodium alginate are most stable at pH=4～10, while alginic acid is precipitated below pH=3. But solutions should not be stored in metal containers, since sodium alginate is incompatible with calcium salts and heavy metals. High concentrations of electrolytes can cause an increase in viscosity until salting-out of sodium alginate occurs.

Both alginic acid dispersions and sodium alginate solutions are susceptible on storage to microbial spoilage which may result in a decrease in viscosity. They should therefore be preserved with an antimicrobial preservative. They may be sterilized by autoclaving or filtration through a 0.22μm filter. Autoclaving may cause a decrease in viscosity.

③ *Safety*　Alginic acid and sodium alginate are generally regarded as nontoxic and nonirritant materials widely used in food products and oral pharmaceutical formulations. The WHO has set an estimated acceptable daily intake of alginic acid and alginate salts used as food additives at up to 25mg/kg body-weight, calculated as alginic acid. Inhalation of alginate dust may be irritant.

(3) Applications in pharmaceutical formulation or technology　Alginic acid and sodium alginate are used in a variety of oral and topical pharmaceutical formulations. In tablet and capsule formulations, they may be used as both a binder and disintegrant at concentrations between 1%～5%. Sodium alginate has also been used in the preparation of sustained release oral formulations since it can delay the dissolution of a drug from tablets and aqueous suspensions.

In topical formulations, alginic acid and sodium alginate are widely used as a thickening and suspending agent in a variety of pastes, creams and gels, and as a stabilizing agent for oil-in-water emulsions. Recently, sodium alginate has also been used for the aqueous microencapsulation of drugs [8, 9], in contrast with the more conventional microencapsulation techniques using organic solvent systems. This method has also been explored to microencapsulate bacteria or living cell due to the mild conditions, as shown in Table 3-7. The formed semipermeable membrane around cells allows the bidirectional diffusion of nutrients, oxygen, therapeutic products and waste while avoids the entrance of immune cells and antibodies at the same time.

Table 3-7. Cell encapsulation approaches based on alginate matrices.[10]

Material	Modification	Cell	Implantation site	Application
Alginate	/	Bone marrow stromal cells, murine derived adipose-tissue stromal cells, islets of Langerhans and PA317/STKJ cells	Subcutaneous space, peritoneal cavity, and under the kidney capsule	Bone and cartilage engineering, diabetes and cancer
Alginate	With RGD	MC3T3-E1, myoblasts and satellite cells	Muscle	Bone regeneration and muscle regeneration
Alginate-PLL-alginate	/	Embryonic stem cells, bone marrow mesenchymal stem cells, islets of Langerhans, chromaffin cells and myoblasts	Peritoneal cavity, subarachnoid space and subcutaneous space	Bone repair and regeneration, chronic neuropathic pain and anemia
Alginate-PLL-alginate	Covalent cross-linking between membranes	Islets of Langerhans and EL-4 thymoma	Peritoneal cavity	Increased stability
Alginate–chitosan	/	Baby hamster kidney cells and human mesenchymal stem cells	Subcutaneous space	Tissue engineering
Alginate–chitosan	Lactose modified chitosan	Chondrocytes	In vitro study	Increased mechanical properties

Therapeutically, sodium alginate has been used in combination with an H2-receptor antagonist in the management of gastroesophageal reflux, and as a hemostatic agent in surgical dressings.

3.3.3 Acacia

(1) Polymer description   Acacia is the dried gummy exudate obtained from the stems and branches of Acacia senegal (Linne) Willdenow or other related species of Acacia (Fam. Leguminosae) which grow mainly in the Sudan and Senegal regions of Africa. Acacia is a complex and loose aggregate of sugars and hemicelluloses with a molecular weight of approximately 240000～580000. The aggregate consists essentially

of an arabic acid nucleus connecting calcium, magnesium and potassium. The hydrolysis of arabic acid will produce sugars of arabinose, galactose and rhamnose.

The manufacture of acacia is described as below. The dried exudates from trees are collected, processed to remove bark, sand and other particulate matter, and graded. Various acacia grades differing in particle size and other physical properties are thus obtained. A spray-dried powder is also commercially available.

(2) Typical properties   Acacia occurs as white or yellowish-white colored thin flakes, spheroidal tears granules or powder with hygroscopicity.

① *Solubility*   Acacia is soluble in water (1:2.7), glycerin and propyleneglycol (1:20). It is insoluble in ethanol (95%). The viscosity of aqueous acacia solutions varies depending upon the source of the material, processing, storage conditions, pH and the presence of salts. Viscosity increases slowly up to about 25% *w/v* concentration and exhibits Newtonian behavior. Above this concentration, viscosity rapidly increases. Increasing temperature or prolonged heating of solutions results in a decrease of viscosity due to depolymerization or particle agglomeration.

② *Stability and storage conditions*   Powdered acacia should be stored in an airtight container in a cool and dry place. Aqueous acacia solutions are subject to bacterial or enzymatic degradation. They may be sterilized by microwave irradiation.

③ *Incompatibility*   Aqueous solutions of acacia carry a negative charge and will form coacervates with gelatin and other substances. Many salts reduce the viscosity of aqueous acacia solutions, while trivalent salts may initiate coagulation. In the preparation of emulsions, solutions of acacia are incompatible with soaps.

④ *Safety*   Acacia is generally regarded as an essentially nontoxic material used in oral and topical pharmaceutical formulations. It is listed in GRAS and included in the FDA Inactive Ingredients Guide for oral preparations. However, there have been a limited number of reports of hypersensitivity to acacia after inhalation or ingestion. Severe anaphylactic reactions have occurred following the parenteral administration of acacia and it is now no longer used for this purpose.

(3) Applications in pharmaceutical formulation or technology   Acacia is mainly used in oral and topical pharmaceutical formulations as a suspending and emulsifying agent, often in combination with tragacanth. Acacia is also used as a tablet binder, which can produce tablets with a prolonged disintegration time. Concentrated aqueous solutions of acacia are used to prepare pastilles and lozenges since they form solid rubbery or glass-like masses on drying.

3.3.4　Xanthan gum

(1) Polymer description   *Structural formula of xanthan gum*:

Xanthan gum is a polysaccharide gum, containing polymer backbone identical in structure to cellulose and trisaccharide side chains, as shown above. The backbone consists of β-D-glucose units linked at the 1 and 4 positions. Each side chain comprises a glucuronic acid residue between two mannose units. The mannose nearest the main chain carries a single acetyl group at C-6 and there is a pyruvate moiety at most of the terminal mannose units, which is prepared as the sodium, potassium, or calcium salt. The resulting stiff polymer chain may exist in solution, as a single, double or triple helix which interacts with other xanthan gum molecules to form complex and loosely bound networks. The molecular weight is approximately 2×10^6.

Xanthan gum is a polysaccharide produced by a pure-culture aerobic fermentation of a carbohydrate with *Xanthomonas campestris*, which is then purified by recovery with propan-2-ol, dried and milled.

(2) Typical properties   Xanthan gum occurs as a cream or white-colored, odorless and free flowing powder.

① *Solubility*   Xanthan gum is soluble in cold or warm water. It is practically insoluble in ethanol and ether. Xanthan gum is available in several different grades with varying particle sizes. Fine mesh grades of xanthan gum are used in applications which have high solubility and dissolve rapidly in water. It is preferable to dissolve xanthan gum in water first and then add the other ingredients in a formulation.

② *Stability and storage conditions*   Xanthan gum is a stable material. The bulk material should be stored in a well-closed container in a cool and dry place. Aqueous solutions of Xanthan gum are stable over a wide pH range (pH=3～12) and temperatures (10～60℃). Solutions are also stable in the presence of enzymes, salts, acids and bases. Xanthan gum solutions are stable in the presence of up to 60% water-miscible organic solvents such as acetone, methanol, ethanol or propan-2-ol. However, above this concentration precipitation or gelation occurs.

③ *Incompatibility*   Xanthan gum is an anionic material, hence it is incompatible with cationic surfactants, polymers and preservatives accompanying with precipitation. Anionic and amphoteric surfactants at concentrations above 15% also cause precipitation of xanthan gum from a solution. Gelation or precipitation occurs with polyvalent metal ions, such as calcium, under highly alkaline conditions. The presence of low levels of borates (< 300ppm) can also cause gelation. This may be avoided by lowering the pH of a formulation to less than pH=5 or by the addition of ethylene glycol, sorbitol or mannitol.

④ *Safety* Xanthan gum is generally nontoxic and nonirritant at the levels employed as a pharmaceutical excipient in oral and topical pharmaceutical formulations. The estimated acceptable daily intake for xanthan gum has been set by the WHO at up to 10mg/kg body-weight. Xanthan gum is listed in GRAS and included in the FDA Inactive Ingredients Guide for oral solutions, suspensions and tablets and for rectal and topical preparations. It is also included in nonparenteral medicines licensed in the UK.

(3) Applications in pharmaceutical formulation or technology Xanthan gum is widely used in oral and topical pharmaceutical formulations as a suspending and stabilizing agent. It is compatible with most synthetic and natural viscosity-increasing agents. Synergistic rheological effects occur when xanthan gum is mixed with certain inorganic suspending agents, such as magnesium aluminum silicate (1:2 ～ 1:9), or organic gums (3:7 ～ 1:9).

Xanthan gum has also been used as matrix for sustained release tablets.

3.3.5 Gelatin

(1) Polymer description Gelatin is a generic term for a mixture of purified protein fractions obtained by partial hydrolysis of animal collagen. The protein fractions consist almost entirely of amino acids joined together by amide linkages to form linear polymers, varying in molecular weight from 15000 to 250000.

Gelatin is extracted from animal tissues rich in collagen such as skin, sinews and bone. It is practical to treat the animal tissues with either acid or alkali. Gelatin obtained from the acid process is called type A, whilst that obtained from the alkali process is called type B. Various grades of gelatin are commercially available with different particle sizes, molecular weights, etc.

In the US, most type A gelatin is obtained from pig skins. This material is washed in cold water for a few hours to remove extraneous matter and is then digested in dilute mineral acid (either HCl, H_2SO_4, H_2SO_3 or H_3PO_4) at pH=1～3 and 15～20℃ until maximum swelling has occurred. This process takes approximately 24 hours. The swollen stock is then washed with water to remove excess acid and the pH is adjusted to pH=3.5～4.0 for the conversion to gelatin by hot extraction.

In the alkali process, demineralized bones or cattle skins are usually used. The animal tissue is held in a calcium hydroxide slurry for a period of one to three months at 15～20℃. At the end of the liming, the stock is washed with cold water to remove as much of the lime as possible. The stock solution is then neutralized with acid (HCl, H_2SO_4 or H_3PO_4) and the gelatin extracted with water in an identical manner to the acid process. The hydrolytic extraction of gelatin solution obtained above is then chilled to form jelled sheets which are dried in temperature-controlled ovens. The dried gelatin is then ground to the desired particle size.

(2) Typical properties   Gelatin occurs as a light-amber to faintly yellow-colored, vitreous and brittle solid. It is practically odorless and tasteless and is available as translucent sheets and granules, or as a powder.

① *Solubility*   Gelatin is soluble in hot water, while it swells and softens in cold water, which can gradually absorb 5~10 times its own weight of water. Gelatin is also soluble in glycerin, acids and alkalis, although strong acids or alkalis cause precipitation. It is practically insoluble in acetone, chloroform, ethanol(95%), ether, and methanol.

② *Gelation*   The gelatin solution exists as a sol at temperatures > 40℃, which forms a jelly or gel on cooling to 35~40℃. This gel-sol system is heat reversible, and the melting point can be varied by the addition of glycerin.

③ *Stability and storage conditions*   Dry gelatin is stable in air, which may be sterilized by dry heat. The bulk material should be stored in an airtight container in a cool and dry place.

Aqueous gelatin solutions are also stable for long periods if stored under cool and sterile conditions. At temperatures above about 50℃ aqueous gelatin solutions may undergo slow depolymerization, and the depolymerization becomes more rapid at temperatures above 65℃. The rate and extent of depolymerization depends on the molecular weight of the gelatin, where material with a lower molecular weight decomposes more rapidly. Gelatin may be hydrolyzed by most proteolytic systems to yield its amino acid components.

④ *Incompatibility*   Gelatin is an amphoteric material and will thus react with both acids and bases. Gelatin will also react with aldehydes and aldehydic sugars, anionic and cationic polymers, electrolytes, metal ions, plasticizers, preservatives and surfactants. It is precipitated by alcohols, chloroform, ether, mercury salts and tannic acid.

⑤ *Safety*   Gelatin is generally regarded as a nontoxic and nonirritant material when used in oral formulations. It is included in the FDA Inactive Ingredients Guide for dental preparations, inhalations, injections, oral capsules, solutions, syrups and tablets, topical and vaginal preparations, and included in medicines licensed in UK. However, there have been rare reports of gelatin capsules adhering to the esophageal lining which may cause local irritation. Hyper-sensitivity reactions, including serious anaphylactoid reactions, have been reported following the use of gelatin in parenteral products.

(3) Applications in pharmaceutical formulation or technology   Gelatin is most frequently used to form either hard or soft gelatin capsules for oral administration. Whilst gelatin is poorly soluble in cold water, a gelatin capsule will swell in gastric

fluid to release its contents rapidly. The USPNF XVII permits gelatin, used to produce hard capsules, to contain various coloring agents, antimicrobial preservatives and sodium lauryl sulfate. Manufacturers may also add a hardening agent, such as sucrose, to hard gelatin capsules. Soft gelatin capsules are formed from an aqueous gelatin solution which contains a plasticizer such as glycerin or sorbitol.

Gelatin is also used for the microencapsulation of drugs, where the active drug is sealed inside a microsized capsule that may then be handled as a powder. Gelatin forms simple coacervates at temperatures above 40℃ with dehydrating agents such as ethanol or 7% sodium sulfate solution.

Low molecular weight gelatin has been investigated to enhance the dissolution of orally ingested drugs. Other uses of gelatin include the preparation of pastes, pastilles, pessaries and suppositories. In addition, gelatin is used as a tablet binder and coating agent, and as a viscosity-increasing agent for solutions and semi-solids. Therapeutically, gelatin has been used as plasma substitute and in the preparation of wound dressings.

3.3.6 Albumin

(1) Polymer description Albumin is a sterile and non-pyrogenic aqueous solution of serum albumin obtained from healthy human donors. It is one of the smallest plasma proteins, comprising about 60% of all the plasma proteins. Albumin contains 584 amino acids, 7 disulfide bridges, and has an isoelectric point of 4.7. The secondary structure of albumin contains about 48% α-helix and 15% β-pleated sheet, with the remainder as a random coil. The molecular weight of albumin is approximately 66500.

Albumin is obtained by the fractionation of blood, plasma, serum, or placentas from healthy human donors. The source material is tested for the absence of hepatitis B surface antigen and HIV antibodies. Separation of the albumin is carried out under controlled conditions, particularly with respect to pH, ionic strength and temperature, so that the final product contains not less than 95% of the total protein as albumin. A suitable stabilizer such as sodium caprylate may then be added. The albumin solution is sterilized by filtration and aseptically filled and sealed in sterile containers. The solution, in its final containers, is heated to 59.5～60.5℃ and maintained at this temperature for 10 hours. The containers are then incubated for not less than 14 days at 30～32℃ or at 20～25℃ for 4 weeks and examined visually for signs of microbial contamination.

(2) Typical properties Albumin appears as brownish amorphous lumps, scales or powder in the solid state. Aqueous albumin solutions are commercially available with different concentration, which are slightly viscous and range in color from almost colorless to amber, depending on the protein concentration. A 4%～5% w/v aqueous solution of albumin is iso-osmotic with serum.

① *Solubility*   Albumin is freely soluble in dilute salt solutions and water. Aqueous solutions containing 40% *w/v* albumin can be readily prepared at pH=7.4.

② *Stability and storage conditions*   Albumin is a protein and is therefore susceptible to chemical degradation and denaturation by exposure to extremes of pH, high salt concentrations, heat, enzymes, organic solvents and other chemical agents. Albumin solutions should be protected from light and stored at a temperature of 2~25℃.

③ *Safety*   Albumin is generally regarded as an essentially nontoxic and nonirritant material, primarily used in parenteral formulations as an excipient. It is included in the FDA Inactive Ingredients Guide (Ⅳ injections) and in parenteral products licensed in UK. Adverse reactions to albumin infusion rarely occur but include nausea, vomiting, increased salivation and febrile reactions. Allergic reactions, including anaphylactic shock can occur. Albumin infusions are contra-indicated in patients with severe anemia or cardiac failure.

(3) Applications in pharmaceutical formulation or technology   Albumin is primarily used in parenteral pharmaceutical formulations as a stabilizing agent for those formulations containing proteins and enzymes. As a stabilizing agent, albumin has been employed in protein formulations at concentrations as low as 0.003% although 1%~5% concentration has also been used.

Albumin is also used to prepare microspheres for experimental drug delivery systems. Albumin has also been used as a cosolvent for parenteral drugs, as a cryoprotectant during lyophilization, and to prevent adsorption of other proteins to surfaces.

Therapeutically, albumin solutions are used parenterally for plasma volume replacement and for treating severe acute albumin loss.

◆ 本节中文导读 ◆

早期使用的药用辅料大都是天然高分子。天然高分子材料来源广泛，品种繁多，按照其化学组成和结构特点可以分为多糖、蛋白等。除了前面提到的淀粉及其衍生物、纤维素及其衍生物，作为药用辅料使用的天然高分子材料还包括：多糖类如壳聚糖、海藻酸、阿拉伯胶、黄原酸胶等；蛋白质类如明胶、白蛋白等。

（1）甲壳素/壳聚糖　甲壳素（chitin）是由 2-乙酰葡萄糖胺以 β-1,4-苷键连接而成的线型多糖，广泛存在于节足动物的翅膀或外壳及真菌和藻类的细胞壁中。壳聚糖（chitosan）是甲壳素经浓碱处理的 N-脱乙酰基衍生物。通常把脱乙酰度>60%或能溶于稀酸的脱乙酰基产物统称为壳聚糖。壳聚糖为白色到乳白色粉末或鳞片状固体，在 95%乙醇、其他有机溶剂及在中性或 pH>6.5 的碱性溶液中几乎不溶。壳聚糖分子量高、线性结构、没有支链，在酸性水溶液中由于氨基质子化而溶解，使多糖分子带正电。壳聚糖的溶解性受分子量、脱乙酰度和溶液中盐离子浓度影响。所得壳聚糖溶液的黏度随其浓度增大、温度下降和脱乙酰化程度增大而增大。壳聚糖的许多性质都与他的聚电解质性质有关，可与金属离子螯合、或与聚阴离子化合物发生静电作用。此外，壳聚糖还具有很好的成膜性、成纤性、通透性、吸附性，以及抗菌、止血等生物学活性。壳聚糖作为保健食品已有商品出售。在药物制剂领域，壳聚糖可应用于凝胶剂、膜剂、小丸、微球、片剂和脂质体的包衣等，还在控释给药、黏膜黏附制剂、速释制剂、结肠给药以及多肽、蛋白和基因药物的输送方面极具潜力。壳聚糖作为药物载体能提高药物吸收，稳定药物成分，增强药物缓释；作为基因载体对 DNA 有一定的保护，能提高基因的表达。

（2）海藻酸（钠/钾/钙）　海藻酸（alginic acid）是褐藻类植物的细胞壁和细胞间隙中自然生成的亲水性胶质糖类化合物，以 1,4-β-D-甘露糖醛酸(M)和 1,4-α-L-古洛糖醛酸(G)为结构单元。海藻酸可溶解在氢氧化钠溶液中，形成黏性溶液；微溶或几乎不溶解于乙醇（95 %）和其他有机溶剂。海藻酸在水中溶胀但不溶解；它能够吸收相当于自身重量 200～300 倍的水。海藻酸不仅可与一价的钠或钾离子结合为海藻酸钠或海藻酸钾，还可以与许多二价和三价阳离子结合，例如：海藻酸钙等。海藻酸用于各种口服和局部给药药物制剂，如用作片剂胶黏剂，各种糊剂、乳膏剂、凝胶的增稠剂和助悬剂，O/W 乳剂的稳定剂。治疗上，海藻酸用作抗酸剂，与 H2 受体拮抗剂结合使用治疗胃食管反流。

（3）阿拉伯胶（acacia gum）　阿拉伯胶是由糖和半纤维素组成的一种复合的、松散的聚集体，其分子量大约为 240000～580000。主要成分是阿拉伯酸的钙、镁、钾盐，还含有阿拉伯糖、半乳糖和鼠李糖。市售阿拉伯胶为白色或黄白色薄片、类球形、颗粒、粉末或喷雾干燥粉末，无臭，味温和。1 份阿拉伯胶可溶解于 20 份甘油、20 份丙二醇、2.7 份水中，几乎不溶解于乙醇（95%）。一般用作乳化剂、稳定剂、助悬剂、片剂胶黏剂、增黏剂等。阿拉伯胶与壳聚糖作为囊材，可通过复凝法制备微囊缓释制剂。

（4）黄原酸胶（xanthan gum） 黄原酸胶为一种高分子量的多糖类胶状物质，主要由 D-葡萄糖和 D-甘露糖单元组成，还含有 D-葡萄糖醛酸，通常以钠、钾或钙盐形式存在。黄原酸胶的分子量大约为 2×10^6。市售黄原酸胶为奶油色或白色、无臭、自由流动的微细粉末。黄原酸胶几乎不溶于乙醇和乙醚；溶于冷水或热水。黄原酸胶是一种稳定的辅料，在酶、盐、酸和碱存在的条件下同样稳定。黄原酸胶在口服和局部药物制剂、化妆品以及食品中广泛用作助悬剂和稳定剂，同时还用作增稠剂和乳化剂。

（5）明胶（gelatin） 明胶是动物胶原蛋白部分水解产物，分子量介于 15000～250000 之间。市售品为几乎无臭无味、透明的薄片、颗粒或粉末。药用明胶按制法不同，经酸水解获得的明胶称 A 型明胶，而经碱水解制备的称 B 型明胶。明胶在乙醇中几乎不溶，在酸和碱中溶解，在水中膨胀和软化。溶胀的明胶颗粒 35℃以上溶解快。0.5%以上的明胶溶液在冷却到 35～40℃时就会形成胶冻或凝胶，这一溶胶-凝胶体系是热可逆的，熔点比凝固点高。明胶广泛应用于各种药物制剂中，最常用来制备硬胶囊或软胶囊。明胶可用作植入药剂中生物可降解的骨架材料，片剂的胶黏剂和包衣材料，溶液剂和半固体制剂的增黏剂。在治疗中，吸收性明胶可以用于制备灭菌薄膜、眼用膜剂、灭菌压缩棉、灭菌棉球和灭菌海绵粉末。明胶海绵有止血作用。

（6）人血白蛋白（human blood albumin） 白蛋白是一种从健康供血者获得的灭菌无热源血清白蛋白制品。白蛋白易溶于稀盐酸和水中，易在极端 pH 条件、高盐浓度、热、酶、有机溶剂和其他化学试剂下发生化学降解和变性。作为辅料，白蛋白主要用于注射制剂，通常被认为是一种基本无毒、无刺激性的物质。白蛋白可用于制备微球和胶囊。白蛋白用作蛋白处方中的稳定剂，注射药物的共溶剂，冷冻干燥过程中的防冻剂。在治疗上，白蛋白溶液可静脉注射用于补充血浆容量和治疗严重的急性白蛋白流失。

References

[1] Hegenbart S. Understanding Starch Functionality. [J/OL]. Food product. Web., 1996. http://www.foodproductdesign.com/articles/1996/01/understanding-starch-functionality.aspx.

[2] Almeida Prieto S, Blanco Mendez J, Otero Espinar F J. Starch-Dextrin Mixtures as Base Excipients for Extrusion-Spheronization Pellets. European Journal of Pharmaceutics and Biopharmaceutics, 2005, 59(3): 511-521.

[3] Loftsson T, Jarho P, Masson M, Jarvinen T. Cyclodextrins in Drug Delivery. Expert Opinion on Drug Delivery, 2005, 2(2): 335-351.

[4] Tiwari G, Tiwari R, Rai A K. Cyclodextrins in Delivery Systems: Applications. Journal of Pharmacy & Bioalled Sciences, 2010, 2(2): 72-9.

[5] Lee B J, Ryu S G, Cui J H. Formulation and Release Characteristics of Hydroxypropyl Methylcellulose Matrix Tablet Containing Melatonin. Drug development and industrial pharmacy, 1999, 25(4): 493-501.

[6] Ratner B, Hoffman A, Schoen F, Lemons J, Biomaterials Science: An Introduction to Materials in Medicine. 2nd Ed. Academic Press, 2004.

[7] Hashimoto M, Morimoto M, Saimoto H, Shigemasa Y, Sato T. Lactosylated Chitosan for DNA Delivery into Hepatocytes: The Effect of Lactosylation on the Physicochemical Properties and Intracellular Trafficking of Pdna/Chitosan Complexes. Bioconjugate Chemistry, 2006, 17(2): 309-16.

[8] Wan L S, Heng P W, Chan L W. Drug Encapsulation in Alginate Microspheres by Emulsification. Journal of Microencapsula tion, 1992, 9(3): 309-16.

[9] Chan L W, Lim L T, Heng P W. Microencapsulation of Oils Using Sodium Alginate. Journal of Microencapsula tion, 2000, 17(6): 757-66.

[10] Murua A, Portero A, Orive G, Hernandez R M, de Castro M, Pedraz J L. Cell Microencapsulation Technology: Towards Clinical Application. Journal of Controlled Release, 2008, 132(2): 76-83.

Chapter 4.

Synthetic Polymers as Pharmaceutical Excipients
合成的药用高分子敷料

4.1 Polymers based on polyvinyl

4.1.1 Polyvinyl alcohol

(1) Polymer description   Structural formula of polyvinyl alcohol:

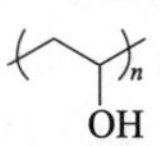

Polyvinyl alcohol (PVA) is a polymer prepared from polyvinyl acetate by replacement of the acetate groups with hydroxy groups. The alcoholysis proceeds most rapidly in a methanol and methyl acetate mixture in the presence of catalytic amounts of alkali or mineral acids, as shown in Scheme 4-1.

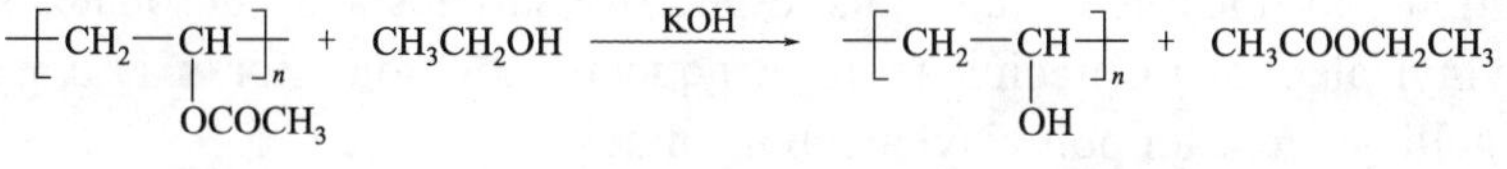

Scheme 4-1. Preparation of PVA from polyvinyl acetate (PVAc)

Various grades of polyvinyl alcohol are commercially available. Two main parameters determine their physical properties, namely the degree of polymerization (n) and the degree of hydrolysis. The pharmaceutical grade is a partially hydrolyzed material, where the polyvinyl acetate is usually about $85\%\sim89\%$ hydrolyzed. The average value of n lies in the range of $500\sim5000$. Commercial grades may be named according to a coding system in which the first two numbers following a trade name indicate the approximate degree of polymerization and the last two numbers refer to the degree of hydrolysis. Taking PVA-1788 as an example, it means that the degree of polymerization is about 1700 and the degree of hydrolysis is about 88%.

(2) Typical properties   Polyvinyl alcohol occurs as an odorless and white to cream-colored granular powder, with melting point at 228℃ for fully hydrolyzed

grades and at 180~190℃ for partially hydrolyzed grades.

① *Solubility*　Polyvinyl alcohol is soluble in hot or cold water and its solubility in water increases as the molecular weight decreases. Effective dissolution of partially hydrolyzed grades requires the dispersion and continued mixing of the solid in cold or tepid water followed by sustained heating at 85~95℃ until dissolved. Polyvinyl alcohol is very slightly soluble in some polyhydroxy compounds, certain amines and amides, and is practically insoluble in aliphatic, aromatic and chlorinated hydrocarbons, esters, ketones and oils.

② *Stability and storage conditions*　Polyvinyl alcohol undergoes slow degradation at 100℃ and rapid degradation at 200℃. It is stable under light exposure. The bulk material should be stored in a well-closed container in a cool and dry place. Aqueous solutions are stable and should be stored in corrosion-resistant containers. For extended storage period, an antimicrobial preservative should be added to polyvinyl alcohol solutions.

③ *Safety*　Polyvinyl alcohol is generally regarded as a nontoxic material. It is included in the FDA Inactive Ingredients Guide for ophthalmic preparations, oral tablets, topical, transdermal and vaginal preparations, and also included in nonparenteral medicines licensed in UK. At concentrations up to 10% it is nonirritant to the skin and eyes. Studies in rats have shown that 5% polyvinyl alcohol aqueous solution injected subcutaneously can cause anemia and infiltrate various organs and tissues. The oral LD_{50} of PVA in rat is > 20g/kg.

④ *Incompatibilities*　Polyvinyl alcohol will undergo typical reactions on secondary hydroxy groups, such as esterification. Polyvinyl alcohol decomposes in strong acids and softens or dissolves in weak acids and alkalis. Incompatibility at high concentration with most inorganic salts, especially sulfates and phosphates will cause 5% polyvinyl alcohol to precipitate from aqueous solution. Borax is a particularly effective gelling agent for polyvinyl alcohol solutions.

(3) Applications in pharmaceutical formulation or technology　Polyvinyl alcohol is a nonionic surfactant and is used as a stabilizing agent for emulsions.

Polyvinyl alcohol is usually used as a viscosity-increasing agent, especially in ophthalmic products, which are generally preferable to have slightly viscous formulations. Polyvinyl alcohol also has desirable lubricant properties which are utilized in many ophthalmic products such as artificial tears and contact lens solutions.

Polyvinyl alcohol is additionally used in the preparation of various jellies which dry rapidly when applied to the skin. It is also used in preparation of sustained release tablet formulations, and in transdermal patches.

Cross-linked polyvinyl alcohol microspheres, used for the controlled release of oral drugs, may be prepared by mixing 30% aqueous polyvinyl alcohol solution with an active drug and glutaraldehyde solution. Moreover, PVA is among embolic materials approved by the FDA[1]. PVA microspheres swelling in an aqueous contrast medium have been used in general embolization to stop uncontrollable bleeding due to cancer, blood vessel malformations and traumatic rupture of blood vessels[2]. Commercial PVA embolic particles such as Contour[TM] and Ivalon have been obtained by the pulverization of a fully saponified PVA sponge.

Crossed-linked polyvinyl alcohol hydrogels may also be formed by repeated freezing and thawing of polyvinyl alcohol solutions. The PVA gels are capable of simulating natural tissue and can be readily accepted into body. Therefore, PVA gels have been used for contact lenses, the lining for artificial hearts and drug delivery carriers, such as for rectal administration[3].

4.1.2　Polymethacrylates

(1) Polymer description　Polymethacrylates are synthetic cationic or anionic copolymers of methacrylic acid, dimethylaminoethylmethacrylates and methacrylic acid esters in varying ratios. They are generally prepared by the polymerization of acrylic and methacrylic acids or their esters, e.g. butyl ester or dimethylaminoethyl ester. Typically, the molecular weight of the polymer is $\geqslant 100000$.

Several different types of polymethacrylates are commercially available, which structural formula is shown below. Three types, namely *Eudragit L*, *Eudragit S*, and *Eudragit L30 D-55* are defined which vary in their methacrylic acid content and solution viscosity. Two additional polymers, namely *Eudragit RL* and *Eudragit RS* are defined as ammonio methacrylate copolymers, consisting of fully polymerized copolymers of acrylic acid and methacrylic acid esters with a low content of quaternary ammonium groups. Detailed information about their components is listed in Table 4-1.

Structural Formula of polymethacrylate：

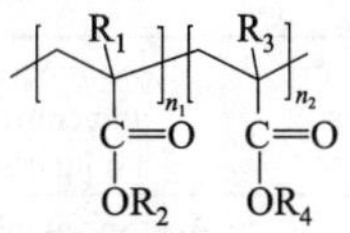

$$
\begin{array}{cc}
R_1 & R_3 \\
\mid & \mid \\
\left[CH_2-C \right]_{n_1} \left[CH_2-C \right]_{n_2} \\
\mid & \mid \\
C{=}O & C{=}O \\
\mid & \mid \\
OR_2 & OR_4
\end{array}
$$

For *Eudragit E*	$R_1, R_3 = CH_3$ $R_2 = CH_2\ CH_2N(CH_3)_2$ $R_4 = CH_3, CH_2\ CH_2\ CH_2CH_3$
For *Eudragit L* and *S*	$R_1, R_3 = CH_3$ $R_2 = H$ $R_4 = CH_3$
For *Eudragit RL* and *RS*	$R_1 = H, CH_3$ $R_2 = CH_3, CH_2CH_3$ $R_3 = CH_3$ $R_4 = CH_2\ CH_2N(CH_3)_3{}^+Cl^-$
For *Eudragit NE 30D*	$R_1, R_3 = H, CH_3$ $R_2, R_4 = CH_3, CH_2CH_3$
For *Eudragit L 30D* and *L 100-55*	$R_1, R_3 = H, CH_3$ $R_2 = H$ $R_4 = CH_3, CH_2CH_3$

Table 4-1. Chemical name and CAS registry number of polymethacrylates.

Chemical name	Trade name	CAS number
Poly(butyl methacrylate, (2-dimethyl aminoethyl) methacrylate, methyl methacrylate) 1:2:1	*Eudragit E 100* *Eudragit E 12.5*	[24938-16-7]
Poly(ethyl acrylate, methyl methacrylate) 2:1	*Eudragit NE 30 D* (*formerly Eudragit 30 D*)	[9010-88-2]
Poly(methacrylic acid, methyl methacrylate) 1:1	*Eudragit L 100* *Eudragit L 12.5* *Eudragit L 12.5 P*	[25806-15-1]
Poly(methacrylic acid，ethyl acrylate) 1:1	*Eudragit L 30 D-55* *Eudragit L 100-55*	[25212-88-8]
Poly(methacrylic acid, methyl methacrylate) 1:2	*Eudragit S 100* *Eudragit S 12.5* *Eudragit S 12.5 P*	[25086-15-1]
Poly(ethyl acrylate, methyl methacrylate, trimethylammonioethyl methacrylate chloride) 1:2:0.2	*Eudragit RL 100* *Eudragit RL PO* *Eudragit RL 30 D* *Eudragit RL 12.5*	[33434-24-1]
Poly(ethyl acrylate，methyl methacrylate，trimethylammonioethyl methacrylate chloride) 1:2:0.1	*Eudragit RS 100* *Eudragit RS PO* *Eudragit RS 30D* *Eudragit RS 12.5*	[33434-24-1]

(2) Typical properties   Different types of polymethacrylates may be obtained as the dry powder, an aqueous dispersion, or as an organic solution, which are summarized in Table 4-2.

Table 4-2. Summary of properties and application of commercially available polymethacrylates (Eudragit, Röhm, Pharma GmbH).

Type	Supply form	Polymer dry weight content	Recommended solvents or diluents	Solubility	Applications
Eudragit E12.5	Organic solution	12.5%	Acetone,alcohols	Soluble in gastric fluid to pH 5	Film coating
Eudragit E 100	Granules	98%	Acetone,alcohols	Soluble in gastric fluid to pH 5	Film coating
Eudragit L 12.5 P	Organic solution	12.5%	Acetone,alcohols	Soluble in intestinal fluid from pH 6	Enteric coatings
Eudragit L 12.5	Organic solution	12.5%	Acetone,alcohols	Soluble in intestinal fluid from pH 6	Enteric coatings
Eudragit L 100	Powder	95%	Acetone,alcohols	Soluble in intestinal fluid from pH 6	Enteric coatings
Eudragit L 100-55	Powder	95%	Acetone,alcohols	Soluble in intestinal fluid from pH 5.5	Enteric coatings
Eudragit L 30 D-55	Aqueous dispersion	30%	Water	Soluble in intestinal fluid from pH 5.5	Enteric coatings
Eudragit S 12.5 P	Organic solution	12.5%	Acetone,alcohols	Soluble in intestinal fluid from pH 7	Enteric coatings
Eudragit S 12.5	Organic solution	12.5%	Acetone,alcohols	Soluble in intestinal fluid from pH 7	Enteric coatings

Continued

Type	Supply form	Polymer dry weight content	Recommended solvents or diluents	Solubility	Applications
Eudragit S 100	Powder fluid	95%	Acetone,alcohols	Soluble in intestinal fluid from pH 7	Enteric coatings
Eudragit RL 12.5	Organic solution	12.5%	Acetone,alcohols	High permeability	Sustained release
Eudragit RL 100	Granules	97%	Acetone,alcohols	High permeability	Sustained release
Eudragit RL PO	Powder	97%	Acetone,alcohols	High permeability	Sustained release
Eudragit RL 30D	Aqueous dispersion	30%	Water	High permeability	Sustained release
Eudragit RS 12.5	Organic solution	12.5%	Acetone,alcohols	Low permeability	Sustained release
Eudragit RS 100	Granules	97%	Acetone,alcohols	Low permeability	Sustained release
Eudragit RS PO	Powder	97%	Acetone,alcohols	Low permeability	Sustained release
Eudragit RS 30D	Aqueous dispersion	30%	Water	Low permeability	Sustained release
Eudragit NE 30D	Aqueous dispersion	30% or 40%	Water	Swellable, permeable	Sustained release, tablet matrix

Eudragit E is cationic polymer based on dimethylaminoethyl methacrylate and other neutral methacrylic acid esters. It is soluble in gastric fluid as well as in weakly acidic buffer solutions (up to approximately pH 5). *Eudragit E* is available as a 12.5% ready-to-use solution in propan-2-ol/acetone(60:40). It is light yellow in color with the characteristic of the solvents. Solvent-free granules contain ≥ 98% dried weight content of *Eudragit E*.

Eudragit L and *S*, also referred to methacylic acid copolymers in the USPNF monograph, are anionic copolymerization products of methacrylic acid and methyl methacrylate. The ratio of free carboxyl groups to the ester is approximately 1:1 in *Eudragit L* and approximately 1:2 in *Eudragit S*. Both polymers are readily soluble in neutral to weakly alkaline conditions (pH=6~7) and form salts with alkalis, thus affording film coats which are resistant to gastric media but soluble in intestinal fluid. They are available as a 12.5% solution in propan-2-ol without plasticizer (*Eudragit L 12.5* and *S 12.5*); and as a 12.5% ready-to-use solution in propan-2-ol with 1.25% dibutyl phthalate as plasticizer (*Eudragit L 12.5P* and *S 12.5P*). Solutions are colorless, with the characteristic odor of solvent. *Eudragit L-100* and *Eudragit S-100* are white free flowing powders with at least 95% of dry polymers.

Eudragit RL and *Eudragit RS*, also referred to ammonio-methacrylate copolymers in the USPNF monograph. They are synthesized from acrylic acid and methacrylic acid esters with *Eudragit RL* having 10% of functional quaternary ammonium groups and

Eudragit RS having 5% of functional quaternary ammonium groups. The ammonium groups are present as salts and give rise to pH-independent permeability of the polymers. Both polymers are water-insoluble, and films prepared from *Eudragit RL* are freely permeable to water, whereas, films prepared from Eudragit RS are only slightly permeable to water. They are available as 12.5% ready-to-use solutions in propan-2-ol/acetone (60:40). Solutions are colorless or slightly yellow in color, and may be clear or slightly turbid. Solvent-free granules (*Eudragit RL 100* and *Eudragit RS 100*) contain more than 97% of the dried weight content of the polymer.

Eudragit RL PO and *Eudragit RS PO* are fine, white powders with a slight amine-like odor. They are characteristically the same polymers as Eudragit RL and RS, containing more than 97% of dry polymer.

Eudragit RL 30 D and *Eudragit RS 30 D* are aqueous dispersions of copolymers of acrylic acid and methacrylic acid esters with a low content of quaternary ammonium groups. The dispersions contain 30% polymer. The quaternary groups occur as salts and are responsible for the permeability of films made from these polymers. Films prepared from *Eudragit RL 30 D* are readily permeable to water, whereas films prepared from *Eudragit RS 30 D* are less permeable to water. Film coatings prepared from both polymers give pH-independent release of active substance. Plasticizers are usually added to improve film properties.

Eudragit NE 30 D is an aqueous dispersion of a neutral copolymer consisting of polymethacrylic acid esters. The dispersions are milky-white liquids with low viscosity and have a weak aromatic odor. Films produced are insoluble in water, but swell and be permeable to water, giving pH-independent drug release.

Eudragit L 30 D-55 is an aqueous dispersion of an anionic copolymer based on methacrylic acid and acrylic acid ethyl ester. The ratio of free carboxyl groups to ester groups is 1:1. Films dissolve above pH 5.5 forming salts with alkalis, which thus afford coatings insoluble in gastric media, but soluble in the small intestine.

① *Stability and storage conditions*   Dry powder polymer forms are stable for at least two years if stored in a tightly closed container at less than 30℃. Above this temperature, powders tend to form clumps although this does not affect the quality of the substance and the clumps can be readily broken up.

Polymethacrylates despersions are sensitive to extreme temperatures and phase separation occurs below 0 ℃. Dispersions should therefore be stored at temperatures of 5～25℃ and are stable for at least one year after shipping from the manufacturer's warehouse if stored in a tightly closed container at the above conditions.

② *Incompatibilities*   Incompatibilities occur with certain polymethacrylate dispersions depending upon the ionic and physical properties of the polymer and solvent. For example, coagulation may be caused by soluble electrolytes, pH changes, some organic solvents and extreme temperature. Dispersions of *Eudragit L 30 D, RL 30*

D, L 100-55 and *RS 30 D* are also incompatible with magnesium stearate.

③ *Safty* Polymethacrylate copolymers are generally regarded as nontoxic and nonirritant materials, which are widely used as film coating materials in oral pharmaceutical formulations. A daily intake of 2mg/kg body-weight of *Eudragit* (equivalent to approximately 150mg for an average adult) may be regarded as essentially safe for humans.

(3) Applications in pharmaceutical formulation or technology Polymethacrylates are primarily used in oral capsule and tablet formulations as film coating agents. Depending on the type of polymer used, films of different solubility characteristics can be produced and utilized for different functions as shown in Table 4-2. *Eudragit E* is used as a plain or insulating film former, which is soluble in gastric fluid below pH 5. In contrast, *Eudragit L* and *S* types are used as enteric coating agents since they are resistant to gastric fluid. Different types are available which are soluble at different pH values, e.g. *Eudragit L* 100 is soluble at pH>6, *Eudragit S* 100 is soluble at pH>7. *Eudragit RL, RS* and *NE 30D* are used to form water-insoluble film coats for sustained release products. *Eudragit RL* films are more permeable than those of *Eudragit RS*, and films of varying permeability can be obtained by mixing the two types together.

Polymethacrylates are also used as binders in both aqueous and organic wet-granulation processes. Larger quantities (5%～20%) of dry polymer are used to control the release of an active substance from a tablet matrix. Solid polymers may be used in direct compression processes in quantities of 10%～50%.

Additionally, polymethacrylate polymers may be used to form the matrix layers of transdermal delivery systems and have also been used to prepare novel gel formulations for rectal administration.

4.1.3 Polyvinylpyrrolidone (Povidone)

(1) Polymer description *Structural formula of povidone*:

Povidone is a synthetic polymer consisting essentially of linear 1-vinyl-2-pyrrolidinone groups. It is characterized by its viscosity in aqueous solution relative to that of water, and expressed as a K-value❶ ranging from 10～120. Approximate molecular weights for different povidone grades are shown in Table 4-3.

---

❶ The K-value is calculated using Fikentscher's equation shown below: $\log z = C\left(\dfrac{75k^2}{1+1.5kc}\right) + K$

where z is the relative viscosity of the solution of concentration c, k is the K-value$\times 10^{-3}$, and c is the concentration in % *w/v*.

Table 4-3. Approximate molecular weights for different povidone grades.

K-value	Approximate molecular weight
12	2500
15	8000
17	10000
25	30000
30	50000
60	400000
90	1000000
120	3000000

(2) Typical properties   Povidone is a fine, white to creamy-white colored, odorless or almost odorless, hygroscopic powder. Povidones with K-values equal to or lower than 30 are manufactured by spray-drying and exist as spheres. Povidone K-90 and higher K-value povidones are manufactured by drum drying and exist as plates. Povidones soften at 150℃.

① *Solubility*   Povidone is freely soluble in acids, chloroform, ethanol, ketones, methanol and water. It is practically insoluble in ether, hydrocarbons and mineral oil. The viscosity of aqueous povidone solutions depends on both the concentration and molecular weight of the polymer employed.

② *Stability and storage conditions*   Povidone darkens to some extent on heating at 150℃, with a reduction in aqueous solution. It is stable to a short cycle of heat exposure around 110～130℃. Steam sterilization of an aqueous solution does not alter its properties. Aqueous solutions are susceptible to mold growth and consequently require the addition of suitable preservatives. Povidone may be stored under ordinary conditions without undergoing decomposition or degradation. However, since the powder is hygroscopic, it should be stored in an airtight container in a cool and dry place.

③ *Incompatibilities*   Povidone is compatible in solution with a wide range of inorganic salts, natural and synthetic resins and other chemicals. It forms molecular adducts in solution with sulfathiazole, sodium salicylate, salicylic acid, phenobarbital, tannin and other compounds. The efficacy of some preservatives (e.g. thimerosal) may be adversely affected by the formation of complexes with povidone.

④ *Safety*   When consumed orally, povidone may be regarded as essentially nontoxic since it is not absorbed from the gastrointestinal tract or mucous membranes. Povidone additionally has no irritant effect on the skin and causes no sensitization. Evidence exists that povidone may accumulate in the organs of the body following intramuscular injection and cause the formation of subcutaneous granulomas at the injection site. A temporary acceptable daily intake for povidone has been set by the WHO at up to 25mg/kg body-weight.

(3) Applications in pharmaceutical formulation or technology   Povidone has

being first used in the 1940s as a plasma expander, although it has now been superseded for this purpose by dextran.

At present, povidone is widely used as an excipient, particularly in oral tablets and solutions. In tableting, povidone solutions are used as binders in wet granulation processes. Povidone is also added to powder blends in the dry form and granulated *in situ* by the addition of water, alcohol or hydroalcoholic solutions. Povidone solutions may also be used as coating agents.

Additionally, povidone is used as a suspending, stabilizing or viscosity-increasing agent in a number of topical and oral suspensions and solutions. The solubility of a number of poorly soluble active drugs may be increased by mixing with povidone.

The molecular adduct formation properties of povidone may be used advantageously in solutions, slow release solid dosage forms and parenteral formulations. The best known example of povidone complex formation is povidone-iodine which is used as a topical disinfectant.

4.1.4 Crospovidone

(1) Polymer description Crospovidone, known as cross-linked povidone, is a water insoluble synthetic cross-linked homopolymer of *N*-vinyl-2-pyrrolidinone. It is prepared by a 'popcorn polymerization' process in an aqueous system with the monomer vinylpyrrolidone and a small quantity of bifunctional monomer (cross-linker).

The corresponding products cannot be named according to a molecular weight (or K-value) due to the insolubility of crospovidone. The products differentiation of crospovidon is done mainly by the particle size distribution and some other physical properties, such as their bulk density and their swelling behavior. The commercial products are available, as listed in Table 4-4.

Table 4-4. Particle sizes of the insoluble Kollidon grades.

Size	Kollidon[①] CL	Kollidon[①] CL-F	Kollidon[①] CL-SF	Kollidon[①] CL-M[②]
< 15μm	—	—	≥ 25%	≥ 90%
< 50μm	≤ 60%	> 50%		—
< 250μm	≥ 95%	≥ 95%	≥ 99%	—

① Registered trademark of BASF group.

② Micronized.

(2) Typical properties Crospovidone is a white to creamy-white, finely divided, free-flowing, practically tasteless, odorless or nearly odorless, and hygroscopic powder.

① *Solubility and swelling property* Crospovidone is practically insoluble in water and most common organic solvents. However, it swells very fast and predictably without forming a gel, which maximum moisture sorption is approximately 60%. The swelling pressure of poured and slightly compacted Kollidon CL powder in water is much higher than that of Kollidon CL-M, Kollidon CL-SF and Kollidon CL-F. The pressure increase per time depends on the particle size distribution and is highest for Kollidon CL, as shown in Table 4-5.

Table 4-5. Swelling pressure and time to reach 90% of the maximum swelling pressure of the insoluble Kollidon grades.

Condition	Kollidon CL	Kollidon CL-F	Kollidon CL-SF	Kollidon CL-M
Swelling pressure/kPa	Ca. 170	Ca. 30	Ca. 25	Ca. 70
Time to reach 90% of the maximum swelling pressure/s	< 10	< 15	< 35	> 100

② *Stability and storage conditions*　Crospovidone is stable. However, it should be stored in an airtight container in a cool and dry place since it is hygroscopic.

③ *Incompatibilities*　Crospovidone is compatible with most organic and inorganic pharmaceutical ingredients. When exposed to a high water level, crospovidone may form molecular adducts with some materials, like povidone.

④ *Safety*　Crospovidone is used in oral pharmaceutical formulations and is generally regarded as a nontoxic and nonirritant material. Short-term animal toxicity studies have shown no adverse effects associated with crospovidone. However, an acceptable daily intake in humans has not been specified by the WHO due to the lack of available data.

(3) Applications in pharmaceutical formulation or technology　Crospovidone is a water insoluble tablet disintegrant used at 2%～5% concentration in tablets. It absorbs water and swells very rapidly, generating a swelling force, high capillary activity and pronounced hydration capacity with little tendency to gel formation. This property makes it useful as a disintegrant in tablets prepared by direct compression or wet and dry granulation methods.

4.1.5　Carbomer

(1) Polymer description　Carbomers are synthetic high molecular weight polymers of acrylic acid cross-linked with either allylsucrose or allyl ethers of pentaerythritol. They contain 56.0%～68.0 % of carboxylic acid (COOH) groups.

A number of different carbomer grades are commercially available which vary in their molecular weight, degree of cross-linking and polymer structure. These differences account for the specific rheological characteristics of each grade. Table 4-6 gives the approximate molecular weight corresponding to three grades of carbomers.

Carbomers designated with the letter 'P', e.g. carbomer 934P, are the only pharmaceutical grades of polymer accepted for oral or mucosal contact products.

Table 4-6. The approximate molecular weight corresponding to three grades of carbomers.

Carbomer	Approximate molecular weight
Carbomer 934	3×10^6
Carbomer 940	4×10^6
Carbomer 941	1×10^6

Carbomers are prepared from acrylic acid copolymerized with approximately 0.75%~2% (w/w) of allylsucrose. The solvent used for the polymerization is normally either benzene, ethyl acetate or a cyclohexane/ethyl acetate mixture.

(2) Typical properties   Carbomers are white-colored, 'fluffy', acidic and hygroscopic powders with a slight characteristic odor. The average particle size of carbomers is at 2~7μm. They decompose at 260℃.

① *Hygroscopicity*   The normal moisture content for carbomer is up to 2% (w/w). A typical equilibrium moisture content at 250℃ and 50% relative humidity is 10% (w/w). The moisture content of a carbomer does not affect its thickening efficiency, but an increase in the moisture content makes the carbomer more difficult to handle, since it is less readily dispersed.

② *Solubility*   Carbomers can be dispersed in water and after neutralization they can form dispersions in ethanol (95%) and glycerin. The acidity for a 0.5% (w/v) aqueous dispersion is at pH = 2.7~3.5, while pH = 2.5~3.0 for a 1% (w/v) aqueous dispersion.

The acidic colloidal solutions of carbomers dispersed in water have low viscosity, which would produce highly viscous gels when neutralized. Carbomer powder should first be dispersed into vigorously stirred water, taking care to avoid the formation of indispersible lumps, then neutralized by the addition of a base. Agents that may be used to neutralize carbomer include: amino acids, borax, potassium hydroxide, sodium bicarbonate, sodium hydroxide and polar organic amines, such as triethanolamine, and lauryl and stearyl amines, which are used as gelling agents in nonpolar systems. Neutralized aqueous carbomer gels are more viscous at pH=6~11. The viscosity is considerably reduced if the pH is less than pH=3 or greater than pH=12, and the viscosity is also reduced in the presence of strong electrolytes. Gels rapidly lose viscosity on exposure to light, but this can be minimized by the addition of a suitable antioxidant.

③ *Stability and storage conditions*   Carbomers are stable, but hygroscopic materials. They may be heated at temperatures below 104℃ for up to two hours without affecting their thickening efficiency. However, exposure to excessive temperatures can result in discoloration and reduced stability. Carbomer powder should be stored in an airtight and corrosion-resistant container in a cool and dry place.

Dry powder forms of carbomer do not support the growth of fungi. However, an antimicrobial preservative such as 0.1% (*w/v*) chlorocresol, 0.1% (*w/v*) methylparaben or 0.1% (*w/v*) thimerosal should be added in unpreserved aqueous carbomer dispersions. The addition of certain antimicrobial preservatives, such as benzalkonium chloride, benzoic acid and sodium benzoate, or high concentrations of preservative can cause a decrease in the viscosity of dispersion. Aqueous gels may be sterilized by autoclaving.

At room temperature, carbomer dispersions maintain their viscosity during storage for prolonged periods of time. Similarly, dispersion viscosity is maintained or only slightly reduced, at elevated storage temperatures if an antioxidant is included or if the dispersion is stored protected from light. Exposure to light causes oxidation, which is reflected in a decrease in dispersion viscosity. However, stability to light may be improved by the addition of 0.05%~0.1% (*w/v*) of a water-soluble UV absorber such as benzophenone-2 or benzophenone-4 in combination with 0.05%~0.1% edetic acid. The UV stability of carbomer gels may also be improved by using triethanolamine as the neutralizing base.

④ *Incompatibilities*　Carbomers are discolored by resorcinol and are incompatible with phenol, cationic polymers, strong acids and high concentrations of electrolytes. Trace levels of iron and other transition metals can catalytically degrade carbomer dispersions. Intense heat may be generated if a carbomer is in contact with a strongly basic material such as ammonia, potassium hydroxide, sodium hydroxide, or strongly basic amines.

⑤ *Safety*　Carbomers are generally regarded as essentially nontoxic and nonirritant materials. There is no evidence in humans of hypersensitivity or allergic reaction to carbomers used topically. Acute oral toxicity studies in animals indicate that carbomer 934P has a low oral toxicity with doses up to 8g/kg being administered to dogs without fatalities occurring.

(3) Applications in pharmaceutical formulation or technology　Carbomers are used mainly in liquid or semisolid pharmaceutical formulations as suspending or viscosity-increasing agents in nonparenteral medicines. Formulations include creams, gels and ointments. And they may also be used in ophthalmic, rectal and topical preparations.

Certain grades of carbomer with a low residual benzene content (such as carbomer 934P or 974P) may additionally be used in oral formulations, as suspentions, tablets, or sustained release tablet formulations. In tablet formulations, carbomers are used as a binder in either direct compression or wet granulation processes. In wet granulation processes, water is used as the granulating fluid. Additionally, oral doses of 1~3g of carbomer have been used as a bulk laxative.

Carbomers are also employed as emulsifying agents in the preparation of oil-in-water emulsions for external use. For this purpose, the carbomer is neutralized partly with sodium hydroxide and partly with a long-chain amine such as stearylamine.

◆ **本节中文导读** ◆

与天然高分子相比，合成高分子辅料大多具有明确的化学结构和分子量，来源稳定，性能优良，可供选择的品种及规格较多。另外，还可以根据给药系统的特点，通过分子设计和新的聚合方法合成具有特定结构的高分子材料，以满足不同类型药物制剂的需要。但是，合成高分子辅料的使用中必须严格控制材料中混杂的未反应单体、残余引发剂或催化剂和小分子副产物等，以避免可能由此产生的生物不相容性问题和与药物的不良相互作用。本节介绍的药用合成高分子辅料主要为已收载入各国药典的聚乙烯类品种，包括：聚乙烯醇、聚丙烯酸树脂、聚维酮、卡波沫等。

（1）聚乙烯醇（polyvinyl alcohol） 聚乙烯醇是水溶性合成聚合物，市售聚乙烯醇分子量范围大约在 20000～200000。因为乙烯醇极不稳定，不存在这种单体，聚乙烯醇主要由聚醋酸乙酯醇解而成。美国药典规定药用聚乙烯醇醇解度为 85%～89%。聚乙烯醇具有极强的亲水性，溶于热水或冷水中；在有机溶剂中不溶。其在水中的溶解性与分子量、醇解度有关，醇解度 87%～89%的产品水溶性最好。聚乙烯醇主要用于局部用药等药用制剂中，如：在乳剂中用作稳定剂；用于人工眼泪、隐形眼镜保养液中起润滑作用；用于口服缓释制剂及透皮贴剂中；用于制备栓塞微球等。

（2）聚(甲基)丙烯酸树脂（polymethacrylates） 聚(甲基)丙烯酸树脂是由丙烯酸和甲基丙烯酸或它们的各种酯（如丁酯或二甲胺乙酯）按不同比例聚合得到的共聚物。不同型号聚(甲基)丙烯酸树脂市售品可能为粉末、水分散体或有机溶液。聚(甲基)丙烯酸树脂主要用作口服片剂和胶囊剂的薄膜衣材料，不同类型聚合物的薄膜的溶解特性不同。如 Eudragit E 用作普通薄膜或隔离层衣料，在 pH<5 的胃酸中溶解；而 Eudragit L 和 S 型则在胃液中不溶，可用作肠溶衣料。

（3）聚维酮（povidone） 聚维酮为乙烯基吡咯烷酮均聚物，分子量范围在2500～3000000。其分子量可用聚维酮水溶液相对于水的黏度来表征，以 K 值来表示，K 值在 10～120 之间。聚维酮吸湿性很强，在酸、氯仿、乙醇、丙酮、甲醇和水中易溶。聚维酮被广泛用作药物辅料，尤其是口服制剂中，如：用作片剂的胶黏剂、作为增溶剂加速难溶药物从固体制剂中的溶出、作为包衣材料；在一些局部用和口服的混悬剂以及溶液中作为助悬剂、稳定剂或增黏剂。口服后，聚维酮不被胃肠道和黏膜吸收，无毒性。

（4）交联聚维酮（crospovidone） 交联聚维酮为水不溶性的 *N*-乙烯基-2-吡咯烷酮交联高分子。交联聚维酮呈白色至乳白色、细分散、自由流动、几乎无味、无臭或稍有气味的吸湿性粉末，几乎不溶于水和常用的有机溶剂，主要用作口服制剂的崩解剂。

（5）卡波姆（carbomer） 卡波姆是丙烯酸与烯丙基蔗糖或与烯丙基季戊四醇醚的交联共聚物，其中含 56 %～68 %的羧基基团（以干品计算），交联度不高，分子量理论上估计在 $7×10^5$～$4×10^6$ 之间。卡波姆具有亲水性，但不溶于水，吸水显著溶胀，形成三维交联的微凝胶，较低浓度时在水中形成酸性的低黏度胶体分散液；中和之后产生高黏度的凝胶。卡波姆主要作为助悬剂或增黏剂应用于液体或半固体的药物剂型中，包括乳膏、凝胶、眼用软膏、直肠和局部制剂。

4.2 Polymers based on polyether

4.2.1 Polyethylene glycol

(1) Polymer description   *Structural formula of polyethylene glycol*:

$$H\left[O\diagup\diagdown\diagup\right]_n O-H$$

Polyethylene glycol (PEG) is a condensation polymer formed by the reaction of ethylene oxide and water under pressure in the presence of a catalyst.

(2) Typical properties   Polyethylene glycol grades 200~600 are liquids whilst grades 1000 and above are solids at ambient temperatures. Liquid grades (PEG 200~ 600) occur as clear, colorless or slightly yellow-colored, and viscous liquids. PEG 600 can occur as a solid at ambient temperatures. Solid grades (PEG≥1000) are white or off-white in color, and range in consistency from pastes to waxy flakes. They have a faint and sweet odor. Grades of PEG 6000 and above are available as free flowing milled powders.

The freezing points and melting points of PEG also vary depending on their molecular weight as listed in Table 4-7.

Table 4-7   The freezing points and melting points of different grades of PEG.

PEG grade	Freezing point	PEG grade	Melting point
PEG 200	$< -65\,^{\circ}\mathrm{C}$	PEG 1000	$37\sim40\,^{\circ}\mathrm{C}$
PEG 300	$-15\sim-8\,^{\circ}\mathrm{C}$	PEG 1500	$44\sim48\,^{\circ}\mathrm{C}$
PEG 400	$4\sim8\,^{\circ}\mathrm{C}$	PEG 2000	$45\sim50\,^{\circ}\mathrm{C}$
PEG 600	$15\sim25\,^{\circ}\mathrm{C}$	PEG 4000	$50\sim58\,^{\circ}\mathrm{C}$
		PEG 6000	$55\sim63\,^{\circ}\mathrm{C}$
		PEG 20000	$60\sim63\,^{\circ}\mathrm{C}$

① *Hygroscopicity*   Liquid polyethylene glycols are very hygroscopic, which hygroscopicity decreases with increasing molecular weight. Solid grades, e.g. PEG 4000 and above, are not hygroscopic.

② *Solubility*   All grades of polyethylene glycol are soluble in water and miscible in all proportions with other polyethylene glycols (after melting, if necessary). Aqueous solutions of higher molecular weight grades may form gels. Liquid polyethylene glycols are soluble in acetone, alcohols, benzene, glycerin and glycols. Solid polyethylene glycols are soluble in acetone, dichloromethane, ethanol and methanol. They are slightly soluble in aliphatic hydrocarbons and ether, but insoluble in fats, fixed oils and mineral oil.

③ *Stability and storage conditions*   Polyethylene glycols are chemically stable in air and in solution. Polyethylene glycols do not support microbial growth, nor do they become rancid. Polyethylene glycols and aqueous polyethylene glycol solutions can be sterilized by autoclaving, filtration or gamma irradiation. Sterilization of solid grades by dry heat at 150℃ for one hour may induce oxidation, darkening and the formation of acidic degradation products. Ideally, sterilization should be carried out in an inert atmosphere. Oxidation may occur if polyethylene glycols are exposed for long periods to temperatures exceeding 50℃. Storage under nitrogen reduces the possibility of oxidation. And oxidation of polyethylene glycols may also be inhibited by the inclusion of a suitable antioxidant.

Generally, polyethylene glycols should be stored in well-closed containers in a cool and dry place. Stainless steel, aluminum, glass or lined steel containers are preferred for the storage of liquid grades.

④ *Incompatibilities*   The chemical reactivity of polyethylene glycols is mainly confined to the two terminal hydroxyl groups, which can be either esterified or etherified. Liquid and solid polyethylene glycol grades may be incompatible with some colors. The antibacterial activity of certain antibiotics, particularly penicillin and bacitracin, is reduced in polyethylene glycol bases. The preservative efficacy of the parabens may also be impaired due to binding with polyethylene glycols. Plastics, such as polyethylene, phenolformaldehyde, polyvinyl chloride and cellulose-ester membranes (in filters) may be softened or dissolved by polyethylene glycols. Migration of polyethylene glycol can occur from tablet film coatings, leading to interaction with core components.

⑤ *Safety*   Polyethylene glycols are generally regarded as nontoxic and nonirritant materials. Polyethylene glycols administered topically may cause stinging, especially when applied to mucous membranes. There are some reports about the hypersensitivity reactions to polyethylene glycols, including urticaria and delayed allergic reactions. The most serious adverse effects associated with polyethylene glycols are hyperosmolarity, metabolic acidosis and renal failure following the topical use of polyethylene glycols in burn patients. Therefore, topical preparations containing polyethylene glycols should be used cautiously in patients with renal failure, extensive burns, or open wounds.

Liquid polyethylene glycols may be absorbed when taken orally, but the higher molecular weight polyethylene glycols are not significantly absorbed from the gastrointestinal tract. Absorbed polyethylene glycol is excreted largely unchanged in the urine. An estimated acceptable daily intake of polyethylene glycols is up to 10 mg/kg body-weight, set by the WHO. In parenteral products, the maximum recommended concentration of PEG 300 is approximately 30% (*v/v*) since hemolytic effects have been observed at concentrations greater than about 40% (*v/v*).

(3) Applications in pharmaceutical formulation or technology   Polyethylene

glycols are water soluble polymers, widely used in a variety of pharmaceutical formulations including parenteral, topical, ophthalmic, oral and rectal preparations.

① Ointment base Polyethylene glycols are stable and hydrophilic substances that are essentially nonirritant to the skin. They are useful as ointment bases. Solid grades are generally employed in topical ointments with the consistency of the base being adjusted by the addition of liquid grades of polyethylene glycol. They do not readily penetrate the skin and can be easily removed from the skin by washing.

② Suppository base Mixture of polyethylene glycols can be used as suppository bases, which shows the following advantages over fats: the melting point of the suppository can be made higher to withstand exposure to warmer climates; release of the drug is not dependent upon melting point; physical stability on storage is better; suppositories are readily miscible with rectal fluids. Disadvantages of using polyethylene glycols are: they are chemically more reactive than fats; greater care is needed in processing to avoid inelegant contraction holes in the suppositories; the rate of release of water-soluble medications decreases with the increasing molecular weight of the polyethylene glycol; polyethylene glycols tend to be more irritating to mucous membranes than fats.

③ Solvent Liquid polyethylene glycols are used as water-miscible solvents for the contents of soft gelatin capsules. However, they may cause hardening of the capsule shell by preferential absorption of moisture from gelatin in the shell. In concentrations up to approximately 30% (v/v), PEG 300 and PEG 400 have been used as the vehicle for parenteral dosage forms.

Polyethylene glycols can also be used to enhance the aqueous solubility or dissolution characteristics of poorly soluble compounds by making solid dispersions with an appropriate polyethylene glycol. Animal studies have also been performed using polyethylene glycols as solvents for steroids in osmotic pumps.

④ Plasticizer In film coatings, solid grades of polyethylene glycol can be used alone for the film coating of tablets or can be useful as hydrophilic polishing materials. Solid grades are also widely used as plasticizers in conjunction with film forming polymers. The presence of polyethylene glycols, especially liquid grades, in film coats tends to increase their water permeability and may reduce protection against low pH in enteric coating films. Polyethylene glycols are useful as plasticizers in micro-encapsulated products to avoid rupture of the coating film when the microcapsules are compressed into tablets.

⑤ Tablet and capsule lubricant Polyethylene glycol grades with molecular weights of 6000 and above can be used as lubricants, particularly for soluble tablets. The lubricant action is not as good as that of magnesium stearate, and stickiness may develop if the material becomes too warm during compression. An anti-adherent effect is also exerted, again subject to the avoidance of over-heating.

⑥ PEGylation[4] Polyethylene glycol polymer chains are usually attached covalently to the target molecule, normally a drug or therapeutic protein to achieve PEGylated derivative. This process of attachment of PEG is named PEGylation, which can "mask" the agent from the host's immune system (reduced immunogenicity and antigenicity), and prolong its circulatory time by reducing renal clearance. PEGylation can also provide water solubility to hydrophobic drugs and proteins. The first approved PEGylated products have already been on the market for 20 years. There exists a variety of drug-delivery systems stabilized with PEG that have received regulatory approval in the USA and/or the EU as listed in Table 4-8.

Table 4-8   Drug-delivery systems stabilized with PEG that have received regulatory approval in the USA and/or the EU.

PEG drug description	Company	Indication	Year of approval
Adagen [(11~17)×5000 mPEG per adenosine deaminase]	Enzon Inc. (USA&Europe)	severe combined immunodeficiency	1990 (USA)
Oncospar (5000 mPEG-L-asparaginase)	Enzon Inc. (USA)/ Rhôn-Poulenc Rorer (Europe)	acute lymphoblastic leukemia	1994 (USA)
Doxil/Caelyx (SSL formulation of doxorubicin)	Alza Corp. (USA) / Schering-Plough Corp. (Europe)	Kaposi's sarcoma, ovarian cancer, breast cancer, multiple myeloma	1995 (USA) 1999 (USA) All 1996 (EU)
PEG-Intron (2×20000 mPEG-interferon-α-2a)	Schering-Plough Corp. (USA&EU)	chronic hepatitis C	2000 (EU) 2001 (USA)
Pegasys (12000 mPEG-interferon-α-2b)	Hoffmann-La Roche (USA&EU)	chronic hepatitis C	2002 (USA&EU)
Neulasta (20000 mPEG-G-CSF)	Amgen Inc. (USA&EU)	febrile neutropenia	2002 (USA&EU
Somavert [(4~6)×5000 mPEG per structurally modified HG receptor antagonist]	Pfizer (USA&EU)	acromegaly	2002 (EU) 2003 (USA)
Macugen (2×2000 mPEG--anti-VEGF--aptamer)	Pfizer (EU)/OSI Pharm. Inc. And Pfizer (USA)	age-related macular degeneration	2004 (USA) 2006 (EU)
Cimzia (2×4000 mPEG--anti-TNFα)	UCB S. A. (USA&EU)	Crohn's disease, rheumatoid arthritis	2008 (USA) 2009 (USA) 2009 (EU)

Notes：mPEG: methoxypoly(ethylene glycol), SSL: sterically stabilized liposome, G-CSF: granulocyte-colony stimulating factor, HG: human growth, VEGF: vascular endothelial growth factor, TNF: tumor necrosis factor.

⑦ Others   Oral administration of large quantities of polyethylene glycols can have a laxative effect. Therapeutically, up to 6L of an aqueous mixture of electrolytes and high molecular weight polyethylene glycol is consumed by patients undergoing bowel cleansing.

In solid dosage formulations, higher molecular weight polyethylene glycols can enhance the effectiveness of tablet binders and impart plasticity to granules. However, they have only limited binding action when used alone, and can prolong disintegration if present in concentrations greater than 5% (*w/w*). When used for thermoplastic granulations, a mixture of the powdered constituents with 10%~15% (*w/w*) PEG 6000 is heated to 70~75℃. The mass becomes paste-like and forms granules if stirred while cooling. This technique is useful for the preparation of dosage forms such as lozenges when prolonged disintegration is required.

Aqueous polyethylene glycol solutions can be used either as suspending agents or to adjust the viscosity and consistency of other suspending vehicles. When used in conjunction with other emulsifiers, polyethylene glycols can act as emulsion stabilizers.

In addition, polyethylene glycols have been used in the preparation of urethane hydrogels which are used as controlled release matrix [5].

4.2.2 Poloxamer

(1) Polymer description *Structural formula of poloxamer*:

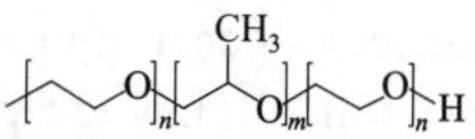

Poloxamers are nonionic triblock copolymers composed of a central hydrophobic chain of polyoxypropylene [poly(propylene oxide)] flanked by two hydrophilic chains of polyoxyethylene [poly(ethylene oxide)], and generally expressed as PEO-*b*-PPO-*b*-PEO. The word "poloxamer" was coined by the inventor, Irving Schmolka, who received the patent for these materials in 1973. Its chemical Name is α-Hydro-ω-hydroxy poly(oxypropylene) poly(oxypropylene) poly(oxypropylene) block copolymer.

Gernerally, poloxamer polymers are prepared by reacting propylene oxide with propylene glycol to form polyoxypropylene glycol firstly. Ethylene oxide is then added to form the block copolymer. Many different poloxamers are commercially available which vary in the molecular weight and the proportion of oxyethylene present in the polymer. A series of poloxamers with greatly varying physical properties are thus available.

Table 4-9 gives the compositions of five poloxamers included in USPNF XVII. The name 'poloxamer' is followed by a number, the first 2 digits of which, when multiplied by 100, correspond to the approximate average molecular weight of the polyoxypropylene portion of the copolymer and the third digit, when multiplied by 10, corresponds to the percentage by weight of the polyoxyethylene portion. For example, Poloxamer 407 indicates a copolymer with a polyoxypropylene molecular mass of 4000 and a 70% polyoxyethylene content.

Table 4-9. Poloxamer grades and their chemical compositions.

Poloxamer	Pluronic®	n	m	Content of Oxyethylene (Percent)	Molecular weight	Physical form
124	L 44 NF	12	20	44.8~48.6	2090~2360	Liqid
188	F 68 NF	80	27	79.9~83.7	7680~9510	Solid
237	F 87 NF	64	37	70.5~74.3	6840~8830	Solid
338	F 108 NF	141	44	81.4~84.9	12700~17400	Solid
407	F 127 NF	101	56	71.5~74.9	9840~14600	Solid

Additionally, there are many of the trade names used for poloxamers. In the USA the trade name Pluronic is used by BASF Corp for pharmaceutical and industrial grade poloxamers, whilst in UK and Europe the trade name Lutrol is used for the pharmaceutical grade material. Take Pluronic F-68 (BASF Corp) as an example, the first digit arbitrarily represents the molecular weight of the polyoxypropylene portion and the second digit represents the weight percent of the oxyethylene portion. The letters 'L', 'P', and 'F' stand for the physical form of the poloxamer, either liquid, paste or flakes.

(2) Typical properties   Poloxamers generally occur as white-colored, waxy, free flowing prilled granules or as cast solids. They are practically odorless and tasteless. Solid poloxamers are free flowing. At room temperature, poloxamer 124 occurs as a colorless liquid. Poloxamers generally contain less than 0.5% (w/w) water and are hygroscopic only at a relative humidity over 80%.

All of the poloxamers are chemically similar in composition, differing only in the relative amounts of propylene and ethylene oxides added during manufacture. Their physical and surface properties vary over a wide range according to a number of different types.

① *Solubility*   Solubility of poloxamer varies according to the type, as shown in Table 4-10.

Table 4-10. Melting point and solubility of poloxamers.

Type	Melting point	Solvent				
		Ethanol (95%)	Propan-2-ol	Propylene glycol	Water	Xylene
Poloxamer 124	16℃	Freely soluble	Freely soluble	Freely soluble	Freely soluble	Freely soluble
Poloxamer 188	52℃	Freely soluble	—	—	Freely soluble	—
Poloxamer 237	49℃	Freely soluble	Sparingly soluble	—	Freely soluble	Sparingly soluble
Poloxamer 338	57℃	Freely soluble	—	Sparingly soluble	Freely soluble	—
Poloxamer 407	56℃	Freely soluble	Freely soluble	—	Freely soluble	—

② *Amphiphilicity and micellation*　Poloxamers are amphiphilic block copolymers, which HLB value varies in the range of 0.5～30, i.e. it is 29 for poloxamer 188. The polyoxyethylene segment is hydrophilic whilst the polyoxypropylene segment is relatively hydrophobic. With an increase of solution temperature or polymer concentration, micellization occurs and a critical micellar concentration (CMC) and a critical micellar temperature (CMT) can be defined [6]. The micelle structure consists of hydrophobic PPO block lying in the micelle core and the PEO block in the corona. The size of PPO blocks influences CMC and the partitioning of hydrophobic moieties in the micelles. Various studies showed that CMC of solutions decreases with increasing temperature.

③ *Cloud point and gelation*　Cloud point of poloxamer is above 100℃ for a 1% (*w/v*) aqueous solution, and a 10% (*w/v*) aqueous solution of poloxamer 188. Aggregation arises as a result of the dehydration of the PPO moieties followed by PEO blocks. Moreover, at high concentration, some poloxamer solutions exhibit a huge increase of viscosity with temperature, leading to a thermoreversible gelation [7, 8]. Generally, this type of behavior is observed in aqueous solutions of concentration ranging from 20% to 30% (*w/w*). Some poloxamer solutions are liquid when refrigerated (4～5℃) but turn into gel form when at room temperature. The formed gel thus is reversible on cooling again.

④ *Stability and storage conditions*　Poloxamers are stable materials. Aqueous solutions are stable in the presence of acids, alkalis and metal ions. The bulk material should be stored in a well-closed container in a cool and dry place.

⑤ *Safety*　Poloxamers are generally regarded as nontoxic and nonirritant materials. Poloxamers are not metabolized in the body. Animal toxicity studies, with dogs and rabbits, have shown poloxamers to be nonirritant and nonsensitizing when applied in 5% (*w/v*) and 10% (*w/v*) concentration, to the eyes, gums and skin. No hemolysis of human blood cells was observed over 18 hours at 25℃, with 0.001%～10% (*w/v*) poloxamer solutions.

(3) Applications in pharmaceutical formulation or technology　Poloxamers are used in a variety of oral, parenteral and topical pharmaceutical formulations. They may be used as wetting agents, in ointments, suppository bases, gels, and as tablet blinders and coatings.

① Emulsifying or solubilizing agents　Poloxamers are nonionic polyoxyethylene-polyoxypropylene copolymers used primarily in pharmaceutical formulations as emulsifying or solubilizing agents. Poloxamers are used as emulsifying agents in intravenous fat emulsions, and as solubilizing and stabilizing agents to maintain the clarity of elixirs and syrups. For example, poloxamer 188 has been used as an emulsifying agent for fluorocarbons used as artificial blood substitutes.

② Wetting agents　Therapeutically, poloxamer 188 is administered orally as a wetting agent and stool lubricant in the treatment of constipation. It is usually used in combination with a laxative such as danthron. Poloxamers may also be used therapeutically as wetting agents in eye-drop formulations, in the treatment of kidney stones and as skin wound cleansers.

③ Hydrogels   Some grades of poloxamer have a unique character of reversible thermal gelation, which have been used as in-situ gelling matrix for protein delivery including IL-2, urease, rat intestinal natrituretic factor and so on. Such in-situ gelling systems have good nondenaturing effects on proteins.

Poloxamer 407 has been used in vehicles for fluorinated dentifrices, eye applications and contraceptive gels. A poloxamer based dental gel product has been used several years for treating patients with sensitive gums and teeth. Moreover, P-407 gel has been shown to possess many favorable characteristics for use as a burn dressing[9].

④ Micelles   It was interesting that poloxamer block polymer (like Pluronic P85) was found to inhibit efflux action of P-glycoprotein, which is linked to multidrug resistance (MDR). The possible reason is that P-glycoprotein efflux requires ATP energy consumption, while Pluronic block polymers may cause significant depletion in ATP levels in MDR cells. Therefore, Pluronic micelles have an additional potential of suppression of MDR as nanocarriers, which is mediated primarily by the monomers[10, 11].

4.2.3   Polysorbates

(1) Polymer description   *Structural formula of polysorbates* 80:

Polysorbates, also named as polyoxyethylene sorbitan fatty acid esters, are a series of fatty acid esters of sorbitol and its anhydrides copolymerized with approximately 20 moles of ethylene oxide for each mole of sorbitol and its anhydrides. Various types of polysorbates are listed in Table 4-11.

Table 4-11. Chemical name, formula, molecular weight and physical form of selected polysorbates.

Polysorbate	Chemical name	Formula	molecular weight	Color and form at 25℃
Polysorbate 20	Polyoxyethylene 20 sorbitan monolaurate	$C_{58}H_{114}O_{26}$	1128	Yellow oily liquid
Polysorbate 21	Polyoxyethylene (4) sorbitan monolaurate	$C_{26}H_{50}O_{10}$	523	Yellow oily liquid
Polysorbate 40	Polyoxyethylene 20 sorbitan monopalmitate	$C_{62}H_{122}O_{26}$	1284	Yellow oily liquid
Polysorbate 60	Polyoxyethylene 20 sorbitan monostearate	$C_{64}H_{126}O_{26}$	1312	Yellow oily liquid

Continued

Polysorbate	Chemical name	Formula	molecular weight	Color and form at 25℃
Polysorbate 61	Polyoxyethylene (4) sorbitan monostearate	$C_{32}H_{62}O_{10}$	607	Tan solid
Polysorbate 65	Polyoxyethylene 20 sorbitan tristearate	$C_{100}H_{194}O_{28}$	1845	Tan solid
Polysorbate 80	Polyoxyethylene 20 sorbitan monooleatee	$C_{64}H_{124}O_{26}$	1310	Yellow oily liquid
Polysorbate 81	Polyoxyethylene (4) sorbitan monooleatee	$C_{34}H_{64}O_{11}$	649	Amber liquid
Polysorbate 85	Polyoxyethylene 20 sorbitan trioleatee	$C_{100}H_{188}O_{28}$	1839	Amber liquid
Polysorbate 120	Polyoxyethylene 20 sorbitan monoisostearate	$C_{64}H_{126}O_{26}$	1312	Yellow liquid

Polysorbates are prepared from sorbitol in a three-step process. Water is initially removed from the sorbitol to form a sorbitan (a cyclic sorbitol anhydride). The sorbitan is then partially esterified with a fatty acid, such as oleic or stearic acid, to yield a hexitan ester. Finally, ethylene oxide is then chemically added in the presence of a catalyst to yield the polysorbate.

(2) Typical Properties   Polysorbates are hydrophilic nonionic surfactants, which HLB value and solubility are summarized in Table 4-12.

Table 4-12. HLB values and solubilities of selected polysorbates.

polysorbate	HLB value	Solubility[①]			
		Ethanol	Solvent Mineral oil	Vegetable oil	Water
Polysorbate 20	16.7	S	I	I	S
Polysorbate 21	13.3	S	I	I	D
Polysorbate 40	15.6	S	I	I	S
Polysorbate 60	14.9	S	I	I	S
Polysorbate 61	9.6	SW	SW	SWT	D
Polysorbate 65	10.5	SW	SW	DW	D
Polysorbate 80	15.0	S	I	I	S
Polysorbate 81	10.0	S	S	ST	D
Polysorbate 85	11.0	S	I	ST	D
Polysorbate 120	14.9	S	I	I	S

① D = dispersible.

Notes: I = insoluble; S = soluble; T = turbid; W = on warming.

① *Stability and storage conditions*   Polysorbates are stable to electrolytes and weak acids and bases. The oleic acid esters are sensitive to oxidation. Polysorbates should be stored in a well-closed container, protected from light, in a cool and dry place.

② *Incompatibilities* Discoloration and/or precipitation of polysorbates occur with various substances, such as phenols, tannins, tars and/or tar-like materials. The antimicrobial activity of paraben preservatives is reduced in the presence of polysorbates.

③ *Safety* Polysorbates are generally regarded as nontoxic and nonirritant materials. However, there have been occasional reports of hypersensitivity to polysorbates following their topical use. The WHO has set an estimated acceptable daily intake for polysorbates 20, 40, 60, 65 and 80, calculated as total polysorbate esters, at up to 25 mg/kg body-weight.

(3) Applications in pharmaceutical formulation or technology Polysorbates are widely used in oral, parenteral and topical pharmaceutical formulations. They may be used as emulsifying agents in the preparation of stable oil-in-water pharmaceutical emulsions. They may also be used as solubilizing agents for a variety of substances including essential oil and oil soluble vitamins, and as wetting agents in the formulation of oral and parenteral suspensions.

◆ 本节中文导读 ◆

本节介绍的药用合成高分子辅料为已收载入各国药典的聚醚类品种，包括：聚乙二醇、泊洛沙姆、聚山梨酯。

（1）聚乙二醇（polyethylene glycol, PEG） 是用环氧乙烷与水逐步加成聚合得到一类水溶性聚醚。其分子量由几百至几千不等，根据分子量由低到高，其性状由黏性液体向糊状、蜡样片状、粉末转变。所有级别的聚乙二醇均溶于水，并且能溶于乙醇、丙酮、二氯甲烷等常用有机溶剂。聚乙二醇无毒、无刺激性，广泛应用于多种药物剂型。如聚乙二醇水溶液可用作注射给药制剂的介质、助悬剂或与其他乳化剂合用增加乳剂稳定性；聚乙二醇在眼用制剂和直肠用制剂中用作栓剂基质；在口服固体制剂中，高分子量聚乙二醇能增加片剂胶黏剂的有效性，影响颗粒塑性，还可用作薄膜包衣聚合物的增塑剂。

（2）泊洛沙姆（poloxamer） 是两端为聚氧乙烯(PEO)、中间为聚氧丙烯(PPO)的三嵌段共聚物，根据其分子量和聚氧乙烯含量的不用，泊洛沙姆有很多品种，可呈液态、半固态和固态。泊洛沙姆是两亲性嵌段共聚物，具有表面活性剂结构特征，易溶于水和一些极性溶剂中。一些泊洛沙姆的水溶液，在浓度高时，会形成凝胶，其胶凝过程是可逆的，具有温度依赖性降低温度，泊洛沙姆会再水化，变成水溶液。泊洛沙姆通常被认为无毒、无刺激性，在体内不被代谢。泊洛沙姆被用于一系列的口服、注射和局部用药物制剂中，如：用作静脉注射脂肪乳的乳化剂，在糖浆剂中用作增溶剂和稳定剂，还可以用作润湿剂、软膏和栓剂基质、凝胶剂和作为片剂的胶黏剂和包衣材料。

（3）聚山梨酯(polysorvates) 也叫聚氧乙烯脱水山梨醇酯（polyoxyethylene sorbitan fatty acid esters），商品名为吐温(Tween)，是一系列聚氧乙烯脱水山梨醇的部分脂肪酸酯，为不同分子量大小的混合物而不是单一的化合物。聚山梨酯为非离子表面活性剂，广泛用作稳定的水包油药物乳剂的乳化剂。聚山梨酯还可用作许多物质的增溶剂，用作口服或非胃肠道混悬剂的润湿剂。

References

[1] Embolic Agents: Choice of Particles for Uterine Artery Embolization for Leiomyomata [cited; Available from: http://www.fibroidoptions.com/agents.htm.

[2] Cha J, Lyoo W, Oh T, Han S, Lee H. Preparation of Syndiotactic Poly(Vinyl Alcohol) Embolic Particles with Radiopacity. Fibers and Polymers, 2014, 15(3): 472–479.

[3] Hassan C and Peppas N, Structure and Applications of Poly(Vinyl Alcohol) Hydrogels Produced by Conventional Crosslinking or by Freezing/Thawing Methods, Biopolymers – Pva Hydrogels, Anionic Polymerisation Nanocomposites. Springer Berlin Heidelberg, 2000: 37–65.

[4] Knop K, Hoogenboom R, Fischer D, Schubert U S. Poly(Ethylene Glycol) in Drug Delivery: Pros and Cons as Well as Potential Alternatives. Angewandte Chemie Internation Edition, 2000, 49(36): 6288–308.

[5] Lin–Gibson S, Bencherif S, Cooper J A, Wetzel S J, Antonucci J M, Vogel B M, Horkay F, Washburn N R. Synthesis and Characterization of PEG Dimethacrylates and Their Hydrogels. Biomacromolecules, 2004, 5(4): 1280–7.

[6] Alexandridis P, Holzwarth J F, Hatton T A. Micellization of Poly(Ethylene Oxide)–Poly(Propylene Oxide)–Poly(Ethylene Oxide) Triblock Copolymers in Aqueous Solutions: Thermodynamics of Copolymer Association. Macromolecules, 1994, 27(9): 2414–2425.

[7] Lenaerts V, Triqueneaux C, Quartern M, Rieg–Falson F, Couvreur P. Temperature–Dependent Rheological Behavior of Pluronic F–127 Aqueous Solutions. International Journal of Pharmaceutics, 1987, 39: 121–127.

[8] Cabana A, Ait–Kadi A, Juhasz J. Study of the Gelation Process of Polyethylene Oxidea – Polypropylene Oxideb –Polyethylene Oxidea Copolymer (Poloxamer 407) Aqueous Solutions. Journal of Couoid and Interfale Science, 1997, 190(2): 307–12.

[9] Patel H R, Patel R P, Patel M M. Poloxamers: A Pharmaceutical Excipients with Therapeutic Behaviors. International Journal of PharmTech Research, 2009, 1(2): 299–303.

[10] Alakhov V, Moskaleva E, Batrakova E V, Kabanov A V. Hypersensitization of Multidrug Resistant Human Ovarian Carcinoma Cells by Pluronic P85 Block Copolymer. Bioconjugate Chemistry, 1996, 7(2): 209–16.

[11] Batrakova E V, Li S, Vinogradov S V, Alakhov V Y, Miller D W, Kabanov A V. Mechanism of Pluronic Effect on P–Glycoprotein Efflux System in Blood–Brain Barrier: Contributions of Energy Depletion and Membrane Fluidization. Journal of Pharmacology and Experimental Therapeutics, 2001, 299(2): 483–93.

Chapter 5.

Novel Synthetic Biodegradable Polymers as Drug Delivery Carrier
新型可生物降解的合成药用高分子材料

5.1 Introduction

The development of biodegradable polymers has attracted increasing interest for the applications in controlled drug delivery systems and in the form of implants and devices for fracture repairs, ligament reconstruction, surgical dressings, dental repairs, artificial heart valves, contact lenses, cardiac pace-makers, vascular grafts, tracheal replacements, and organ regeneration. Examples are the work done on polyesters, poly(orthoesters), poly(anhydrides), poly(phosphazenes), polyamides and so on.

Generally speaking, the term "degradation" refers to a chemical process, resulting in the cleavage of covalent bonds. Hydrolysis is the most common chemical process by which polymers degrade, and degradation can also occur via oxidative and enzymatic mechanisms.

A biodegradable therapeutic agent delivery system has several additional advantages: ①eliminating the need to remove the drug depleted device; ②having greater flexibility in release rate; ③depending less on drug characteristics in comparison with diffusion-controlled systems. However, there are more stringent requirements for them in terms of their biocompatibility. In addition to the potential problem of toxic contaminants leaching from the material, one must also consider the potential toxicity of the degradation products and subsequent metabolites.

By 1999, only five distinct synthetic and degradable polymers have been approved for use in narrow range of clinical applications. These polymers are poly(lactic acid), poly(glycolic acid), polydioxanone, polycaprolactone and poly(PCPP-SA anhydride). In these cases, an important option to consider in their selection is the chemical structure of the polymer (degree of hydrophobicity, covalent bonds between monomers, etc.), because the degradation speed, the degradation condition, and the rate and site of drug release can be modulated in accordance with chemical structure of biodegradable polymers.

The purpose of this chapter is to review the structure, properties, and applications of the different biodegradable polymers actually available[1] and to describe some of their release kinetics, safety, and biocompatibility considerations.

5.2 Polymers based on polyester

5.2.1 Poly(lactic acid) and poly(lactic–*co*–glycolic acid) copolymers

(1) Polymer description   Poly(lactic acid) and poly(lactic-*co*-glycolic acid) copolymers are currently the most widely investigated and most commonly used synthetic, degradable polymers.   Poly(lactic acid) is also called polylactide (*Abbr.* PLA). Poly(lactic-*co*-glycolic acid) copolymers are linear polyesters of lactide and glycolide (*Abbr.* PLGA). Their structures are shown below. These polymers were originally developed as biodegradable sutures and were approved because they degrade to the natural metabolites L-lactic acid and glycolic acid. Because lactic acid has a chiral center, poly(lactic acid) can exist in four stereoisomeric forms, poly(L-lactic acid), poly(D-lactic acid), meso-poly(D,L-lactic acid) and the racemic poly (D,L-lactic acid).

Structural formula of poly (lactic acid) and poly (glycolic acid):

$$\left[\!\!\begin{array}{c} CH_3\ \ O\\ |\ \ \ \ \ \| \\ O—CH—C \end{array}\!\!\right]_n \qquad \left[\!\!\begin{array}{c} O\\ \| \\ O—CH_2—C \end{array}\!\!\right]_n$$

Poly(lactic acid)　　　　　Poly(glycolic acid)

Low molecular weight poly(lactic acid) and poly(lactic-*co*-glycolic acid) copolymers (<3000) can be synthesized by direct polycondensation of lactic or glycolic acid using phosphoric acid, p-toluene sulfonic acid and antimony trifluoride as acid catalysts.

Linear lactide- and glycolide-based polymers are most commonly synthesized by ring-opening melt polymerization of lactide or/and glycolide at $140\sim180\,^\circ\mathrm{C}$ for $2\sim10$ h using a catalyst. Stannous octoate is the commonly used polymerization catalyst because it has been approved by FDA as a food stabilizer. A hypothetical mechanism of the ring-opening polymerization of lactide using a tin catalyst was suggested in the literature[2]. In this mechanism, Lewis acid character of the tin catalyst activates the ester carbonyl group in the dilactone (a, in Scheme 5-1). The activated species reacts with the alcohol initiator to form an unstable intermediate, which opens to the ester alcohol (b, in Scheme 5-1). The propagation reaction proceeds by tin catalyst activation of another dilactone carbonyl group and reaction with the hydroxyl end group. Lauryl alcohol is generally added to control the molecular weight of the polymer. Polymers with a molecular weight as high as 500000 can be obtained by the melt process when high purity monomers (>99.9%) are used. On the basis of this mechanism, branched lactide polymers can be prepared from the polymerization of lactide with various polyol molecules as branching agents. Star poly(ethylene oxide)-polylactide copolymers in a spherical form have been obtained from the block copolymerization of lactic acid on the end groups of three or four arm poly(ethylene oxide) molecules.

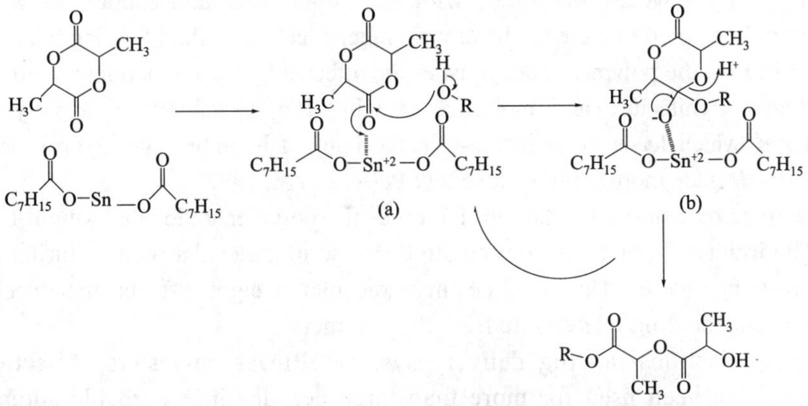

Scheme 5-1. Hypothetical mechanism of the ring-opening polymerization
of lactide using tin octoate as catalyst.

(2) Typical properties The optically active homopolymers poly(D-lactic acid) (PDLA) and poly(L-lactic acid) (PLLA) are semicrystalline materials, whereas the racemic PDLLA is always amorphous. Racemic PDLLA and PLLA have T_g of 57°C and 56°C, respectively, but PLLA is highly crystalline with a T_m of 170°C. PGA is highly crystalline, which has a very high tensile strength (70~140MPa) and modulus of elasticity (about 7000MPa) in its highly crystalline form.

① *Solubility* Poly(lactic acid) and its copolymers with less than 50% glycolic acid content are soluble in common solvents such as chlorinated hydrocarbons, tetrahydrofuran and ethyl acetate. Poly(glycolic acid) (PGA) is insoluble in common solvents, but soluble in hexafluoroisopropanol and hexafluoroacetone sesquihydrate.

② *Degradation*[3] The degradation of the polymeric backbone of PLA is predominantly controlled by simple hydrolysis. The factors that may affect the polylactide degradation include chemical and configurational structure, molecular weight and distribution, crystallinity, fabrication conditions, site of implantation and degradation conditions. Lower molecular weight polymers degraded faster than higher molecular weight polymers. The degradation of semicrystalline PLA proceeds in two phases: in the first phase the amorphous regions are hydrolyzed, and then the crystalline regions in the second. Overall, the degradation process of PLA is a little complex, which can be divided into four steps. In step 1, water diffuses into the polymer and ester bond cleavage starts. In step 2, differentiation between the surface and interior begins, with a drastic decrease in molecular weight in the inner part of the matrix. In step 3, low-molecular-weight oligomers begin to diffuse through the thinning outer layer, and when the molecular weight of these oligomers is low enough to allow solubilization in the medium, weight loss begins. In the final step 4, slow erosion of the polymer shell takes place. It was reported that PLA lost about 50% of its mechanical strength after 18 weeks in buffer, with no weight loss until about 30 weeks of hydrolysis. It is noted that the acidic environment accelerates the PLA degradation.

For PLGA, the polymer characteristics are affected by the co-monomer composition, the polymer architecture and molecular weight. The crystallinity is rapidly lost in copolymers, which leads to an increase in the rates of hydration and hydrolysis. 50:50 copolymers degrade more rapidly than either PGA or PLA.

Sterilization using γ-irradiation decreases the polymer molecular weight by 30 to 40%. The irradiated polymers continue to decrease in molecular weight during storage at room temperature. This decline in molecular weight affects the mechanical properties and the drug release rate from the polymers.

(3) Applications in drug delivery system　Linear polyesters of lactide and glycolide have been used for more than three decades in absorbable sutures and absorbable drug delivery systems. They have been used for the delivery of steroids, anticancer agents, peptides and proteins, antibiotics, anesthetics, and vaccines, where the formulation contains implant, injectable microspheres and so on. Examples of commercialized device based on poly(lactic-*co*-glycolic acid) copolymers are listed in Table 5-1. Of these, the highest commercial success is Zoladex®, which releases a luteinizing hormone releasing hormone (LHRH) analog, goserelin for the treatment of prostate cancer. Repeated administration at 1-, or 3-month intervals is a common palliative treatment for prostate cancer in patients who are at a poor surgical risk.

Table 5-1.　Examples of commercialized device based on poly(lactic-*co*-glycolic acid) copolymers.

Trade name	Device form	Drug
Superfact® Depot	Strand	Buserilin
Zoladex®	Strand	Goserilin
Decapeptyl Depot®	Microspheres	Triptorelin
Enantone LP®	Microspheres	Leuprorelin
Somatulin LP®	Microspheres	Lanreotide
Parlodel LAR®	Microspheres	Bromocriptine
Sandostatin-LAR®	Microspheres	Ocreotide
Eligard 7.5®	Solution of polymer and drug in NMP	Leuprolide Acetate
Nutropin®	Microspheres	Recombinant Human Growth Hormone
Lupron®	Microspheres	Leuprolide Acetate

A triblock copolymer based on poly(lactic-*co*-glycolic acid) and poly(ethylene glycol) copolymer is under development of the trade-name ReGel®. It is of more interest as biodegradable thermogelling materials for injectable gelling systems. When the block lengths and relative amounts are correctly chosen, the obtained material is soluble in water at room temperature and forms a firm gel at body temperature[4]. The biodegradable thermogelling copolymer hydrogels have great applicative potential in areas such as sustained drug release, gene delivery and tissue engineering. A formulation of paclitaxel in ReGel® is known as OncoGel® for local injection, which is designed to provide high concentrations of paclitaxel at the tumour site while minimising exposure to other organs. A dose-escalation study of Phase II is ongoing for oesophageal cancer and Phase I/II for primary brain cancer [5, 6]. In non-clinical models OncoGel™ has been shown to continuously release paclitaxel for up to six weeks to provide concentrations of the drug several orders of magnitude higher at the tumour site than in the blood. In a small Phase II study of OncoGel™ in patients with late stage inoperable oesophageal cancer, 70% of patients had a reduction in tumour volume when OncoGel™ was used in combination with radiotherapy.

5.2.2 Polycaprolactone

(1) Polymer description   Polycaprolactone is also one of degradable polyesters commonly used in drug delivery systems and medical devices. Poly(ε-caprolactone) (PCL) can be synthesized from the anionic, cationic, and coordination polymerization of ε-caprolactone using different types of initiators. The anionic method of polymerization is most useful for the synthesis of low molecular weight hydroxyterminated oligomers and polymers. High molecular weight homopolymers and random copolymers with lactides and other lactones were obtained using coordination catalysts such as di-n-butyl zinc, stannous octoate and so on. Polymerization occurs at 120 ℃ under argon to yield polymers with a narrow molecular weight distribution ($M_w/M_n = 1.1$) and molecular weights above 50000. The polymerizing mechanism is similar to that of polylactide as shown in Scheme 5-2.

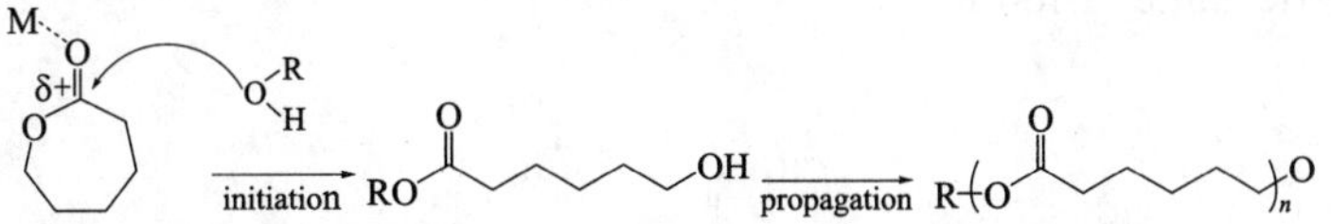

Scheme 5-2. Polymerization of ε-caprolactone using coordination catalysts.

(2) Typical properties   The polycaprolactone homopolymer melts at 59~64℃ with a T_g of −60℃. Copolymerization with lactide increases the T_g with the increase of the lactide content in the polymer. Polycaprolactone is a semicrystalline polymer. The crystallinity of PCL decreases with the increase in polymer molecular weight: the polymer of 5000 is 80% crystalline, whereas the polymer of 60000 is 45% crystalline.

① *Solubility*   Polycaprolactone is soluble in chlorinated and aromatic hydrocarbons, cyclohexanone, and 2-nitropropane, and it is insoluble in aliphatic hydrocarbons, diethyl ether and alcohols.

② *Biodegradation*   Like the lactide polymers, PCL and its copolymers degrade both in vitro and in vivo by bulk hydrolysis, with the degradation rate affected by the size and shape of the device and the additives. Complete degradation and elimination of PCL homopolymers may last for 2 to 4 years. The degradation rate is significantly increased by copolymerization or blending with lactide and glycolide. The rate of degradation can be increased also by the addition of oleic acid or tertiary amines to the polymer, which catalyzes the chain hydrolysis.

③ *Safty*   Polycaprolactone and its monomer ε-caprolactone are currently regarded as nontoxic and tissue-compatible materials.

(3) Applications in drug delivery system or medical device   Polycaprolactone can be used in drug delivery devices that remain active for over one year due to its degradation behavior. The capronor system[●], a one-year implantable contraceptive device has become commercially available in Europe and the US. Capronor is a single-capsule, subdermal contraceptive made of biodegradable PCL, which releases levonorgestrel over a 12- to 18-month period[7]. Additionally, polycaprolactone is already in clinical use as a degradable staple for wound closure.

5.2.3   Poly(*β*–hydroxybutyrate)

(1) Polymer description   Poly(*β*-hydroxybutyrate) (PHB) is a representative polyesters made by a controlled bacterial fermentation. The producing organism occurs naturally. An optically active copolymer of 3-hydroxybutyrate (3HB) and 3-hydroxyvalerate (3HV) as shown in Scheme 5-3 has been produced from propionic acid or pentanoic acid by Alcaligenes eutrophus. The copolymer compositions (0 to 95 mol% 3HV content) can be controlled by the composition of the carbon sources. PHB and its copolymers with up to 30% 3-hydroxyvaleric acid are now commercially available under the trade name "Biopol".

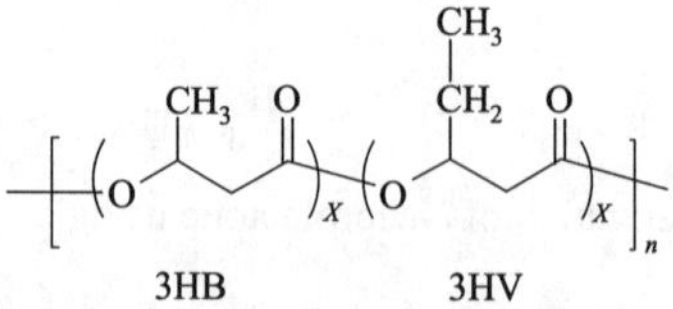

Scheme 5-3. Structural formula of copolymer comprised of 3HB and 3HV.

(2) Typical properties   PHB homopolymer is very crystalline and brittle, whereas the copolymers of PHB with hydroxyvaleric acid are less crystalline, more flexible and more readily processable. The polymers are characterized as having a high molecular

---

❶ Capronor is a registered trademark of the Research Triangle Institute, Research Triangle Park, North Carilina.

weight (M_w >100000; [η] > 3dL/g) with a narrow polydispersity and a crystallinity of around 50%. The melting point depends on the polymer composition. P(3HB) homopolymer melts at 177℃ with a T_g at 9℃, and the 1:1 copolymer with 3HV melts at 91℃.

PHB and its copolymers can be degraded by soil bacteria but relatively stable under physiological conditions. PHB degrades to D-3-hydroxybutyric acid in vivo, which is a normal constituent of human blood. However, it was reported that the polymer typically retained 80% of its original stiffness over 500 days on in vivo degradation and required several years for complete resorption in vivo[8]. The rate of degradation can be modified slightly by varying the copolymer composition within a relatively narrow window. Copolymers having a higher fraction of 3HV and low molecular weight polymers are more susceptible to hydrolysis.

(3) Applications in drug delivery system   PHB and the copolymers have been considered in biomedical applications as controlled drug release carriers, sutures, artificial skin, vascular grafts and so on. PHB is attractive for orthopedic applications because of its slow degradation time.

5.3   Other biodegradable polymers

5.3.1   Poly(orthoesters)

(1) Polymer description   Poly(orthoesters) are a family of synthetic, degradable polymers. There are three major types of poly(ortho esters). The first type are those prepared by a transesterification of 2,2'-dimethoxyfuran with a diol as shown in Scheme 5-4 . The general synthesis involved the heating of the reaction mixture to 110～115℃ for about 1.5～2 h and then further heated at 180℃ and 1.33Pa for 24 h.

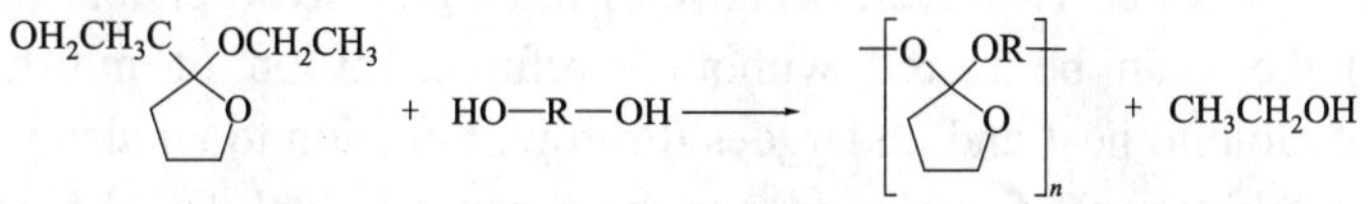

Scheme 5-4. Synthesis of poly(ortho esters) Ⅰ.

The next generation of poly(ortho esters) are based on an acid-catalyzed addition of diols with diketene acetals as shown in Scheme 5-5.

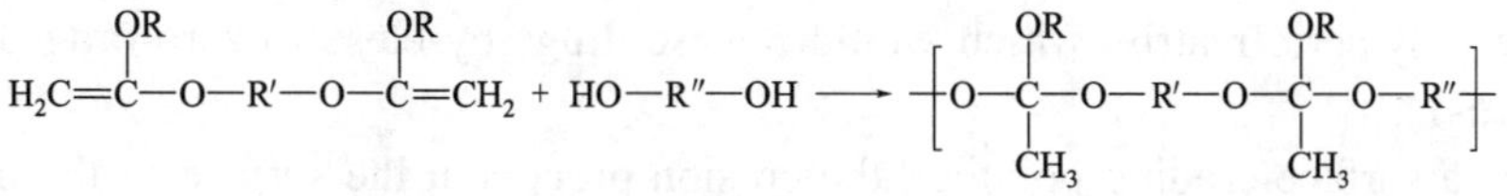

Scheme 5-5. Synthesis of poly(ortho esters) Ⅱ.

The molecular weight of poly(orthoesters) are significantly dependent on the type of diol and catalyst used for synthesis. A linear, flexible diol like 1,6-hexanediol will give molecular weights greater than 200000, whereas bisphenol A in the presence of catalyst will give molecular weight only around 10000.

(2) Typical properties   The properties of poly(orthoesters) can be controlled to a large extent by the choice of the diols used in the synthesis. For example, mechanical properties of the linear poly(orthesters) vary over a large range by selecting various compositions of diols. It was shown that the glass transition temperature of poly(orthoesters) II prepared from DETOSU [3,9-bis(ethylidene-2,4,8,10-tetraoxaspiro (5,5)undecane)] could be varied from 25℃ to 110℃ by simply changing the amount of 1,6-hexanediol in trans-1,4-cyclohexane dimethanol from 100 to 0%[9]. There seems to be a linearly decreasing relationship between the T_g and the percentage of 1,6-hexanediol.

① *Biodegradation*   The primary mechanism for the degradation of poly (orthoesters) is via hydrolysis. As shown in Scheme 5-6, the hydrolysis of poly(orthoesters) I in water generates γ-hydroxybutyric acid, which would accelerate polymer degradation (autocatalytic effect). Incorporating a base into the matrix can stabilize the interior of the matrix. This phenomenon that the hydrolysis of orthoester linkages is sensitive to the medium has been utilized as an advantage in designing the orthoester-based delivery systems.

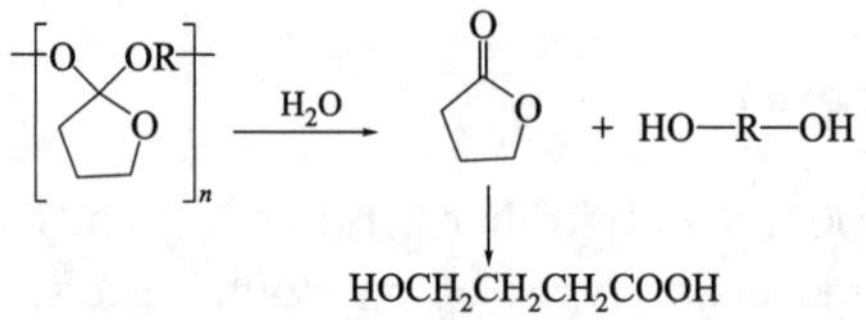

Scheme 5-6. Hydrolysis of poly(orthoesters) I .

② *Stability and storage conditions*   The orthoester linkage is inherently unstable in the presence of water. However, because of the highly hydrophobic nature of poly (ortho-esters) they can be stored without careful exclusion of moisture. But the polymer is unstable to heat and undergoes disproportionation to an alcohol and ketene acetal. The combination of moisture and heat can be fatal for the processing of poly(orthoesters), which are designed to erode within days.

(3) Applications in drug delivery system   Poly(orthoesters) has been developed as a bioerodible and subdermally implantable polymer. Devices made of poly (orthoesters) can erode by "surface erosion" if appropriate excipients are incorporated into the polymeric matrix, which would release drugs by close to zero-order kinetics (Figure 5-1).

For a surface-eroding polymer, the erosion process at the surface of the polymer should be much faster than in the interior of the device. Hence, the polymeric devices with an acid-sensitive orthoester linkage in the backbone could provide a surface-eroding

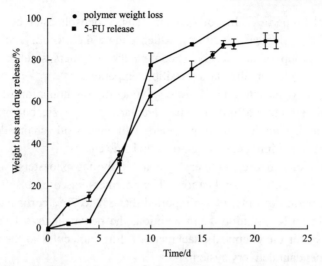

Figure 5-1. Polymer weight loss (•) and 5-fluorouracil (5-FU) release (■) from
a polyorthoester (Drug loading 20 wt%, 0.05 M phosphate buffer, pH 7.4, 37 ℃).[10]

polymer if the interior of the matrix is buffered with basic salts. This approach has been
used in the temporal controlled release of tetracycline over a period of weeks in the
treatment of periodontal disease and the in controlled delivery of contraceptive steroids
for at least 6 months.

5.3.2 Poly(phosphate esters)

(1) Polymer description   Poly(phosphoesters) were synthesized from the reaction
of ethyl or phenyl phosphorodichloridates and various dialcohols including bisphenol A
and poly(ethylene glycol) of various molecular weights, as shown in Scheme 5-7.
Interfacial condensation using bisphenol A as comonomer could yield polymers with an
average molecular weight of 30000~50000.

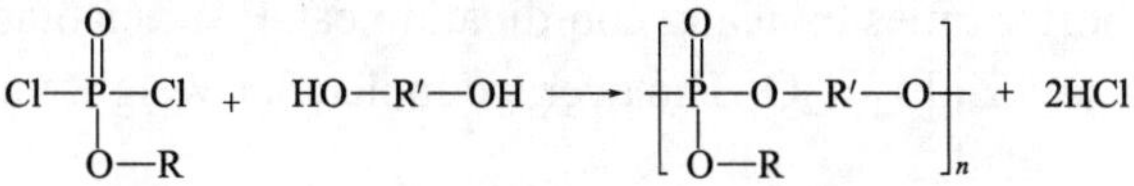

Scheme 5-7. Synthesis of poly(phosphoesters).

In addition, Leong et al[11]. recently designed a new biodegradable material
poly(phosphoester-urethanes) by introducing phosphoester linkage in poly(urethane)
for controlled release applications. Poly(phosphoester-urethanes) are obtained by the
reaction of polydiols and di-isocyanates with phosphates as chain extenders.
Introduction of phosphoester linkage does not change the mechanical properties
inherent in the poly(urethanes) and provides an excellent biodegradation.

(2) Typical properties　In poly(phosphoesters), phosphoester bonds are readily cleaved under physiological conditions, which endow them biodegradation. And the flexible P-O-C group in the backbone confers the polymers solubility in common organic solvents and lowers the glass transition temperature.

Moreover, poly(phosphoesters) is attractive as the manipulation of the backbone or the side-chain structure afford an expansive variety of physicochemical properties. For example, the degradation rate of polymers with phenyl side chains degraded much slower than those containing ethyl or ethoxyethyl side chains.

(3) Applications in drug delivery system　Poly(phosphoesters) is an excellent biomaterial for drug delivery applications. The polymers based on bisphenol A release drug for a long period of time. It was reported that 8% to 20% cortisone was released after 75 days in buffer solution[12]. In addition, the pentavalency of the phosphorus atom also allows for the chemical attachment of drug molecules to the polymer for a biodegradable pendant delivery system.

5.3.3　Polyanhydrides

(1) Polymer description　Polyanhydrides are a class of biodegradable polymers characterized by anhydride bonds connecting repeat units of the polymer backbone chain. There are three main classes of polyanhydrides: aliphatic, unsaturated and aromatic, determined by the R groups as shown below.

Polyanhydrides can be prepared by melt/solution polycondensation or ring-opening polymerization. Melt polycondensation is achieved by simply refluxing the diacid monomer with acetic anhydride for a specified length of time to generate prepolymer. Polyanhydrides are obtained subsequently by heating the prepolymer under vacuum to eliminate the acetic anhydride. Significantly higher molecular weights were obtained in shorter times by using coordination catalysts such as cadmium acetate, earth metal oxides, and $ZnEt_2 \cdot H_2O$. The average molecular weight varying from 90000 to 240000 can be obtained.

(2) Typical properties　Almost all polyanhydrides show some degree of crystallinity as manifested by their crystalline melting points. The homopolymers are highly crystalline and the crystallinity of the copolymers is determined by the monomer of highest concentration. Copolymers with a composition close to 1:1 are essentially amorphous.

The melting points of aromatic polyanhydrides are much higher than those of the aliphatic polyanhydrides. The melting point of the aliphatic aromatic copolyanhydrides is proportional to the aromatic content.

① *Solubility*　The majority of polyanhydrides dissolves in solvents such as dichloromethane and chloroform. However, the aromatic polyanhydrides display much lower solubility than the aliphatic polyanhydrides.

② *Biodegradation*　Anhydride linkage is extremely susceptible to hydrolysis in presence of moisture to generate the dicarboxylic acids. Aliphatic polyanhydrides degrade within days, whereas some aromatic polyanhydrides degrade over several years. The aliphatic-aromatic copolymers usually show intermediate degradation rate depending on the monomer composition. Many polyanhydrides degrade by surface erosion without the need to incorporate other excipients into the device formulation due to their high rate of degradation.

③ *Incompatibility*　Polyanhydrides are highly reactive, which will react with drugs containing free amino groups or other nucleophilic functional groups, especially during high-temperature processing.

(3) Applications in drug delivery system　Polyanhydrides were developed as the surface-eroding matrix for applications in controlled drug delivery. Drug loaded devices made of polyanhydrides can be prepared by compression molding or microencapsulation. A wide type of drugs and proteins including insulin, bovine growth factors, angiogensis inhibitors (e.g., heprin and cortisone), enzymes (e.g., alkaline phosphatase and β-galactosidase), and anesthetics have been incorporated into polyanhydrides matrices for investigation. The first polyanhydride-based drug delivery system to enter clinical use is for the delivery of chemotherapeutic agents. It is BCNU(bis-chloroethylnitrosourea)-loaded implant for the treatment of glioblastoma multiformae, a universally fatal brain cancer [13]. The implant is made of the polyanhydride derived from bis-p-carboxyphenoxypropan and sebacic acid, which received FDA regulatory approval in the fall of 1996.

5.3.4　Poly(amino acids)

(1) Polymer description　Amide-based polymers are polymers composed of amino acids, which are promising candidates in biomedical applications due to their degradation to natural endogenetic amino acids. Except for the natural proteins such as collagen, gelatin and albumin mentioned previously, we focus on the synthetic poly(amino acids) and "pseudo"- poly(amino acids) here.

Poly(aspartic acid), poly(glutamic acid) and poly(lysine) and their copolymers with various amino acids are the most commonly investigated poly(amino acids) used in medicine. These poly(amino acids) are prepared normally by the polymerization of α-amino acid-N-carboxyanhydrides (NCAs) (Scheme 5-8).

Pseudo-poly(amino acids) refer to some backbone-modified poly(amino acids) based on amino acids, which were first suggested by Kohn and Langer in 1987[14], who prepared a polyester from *N*-protected trans-4-hydroxy-L-proline, and a poly (iminocarbonate)

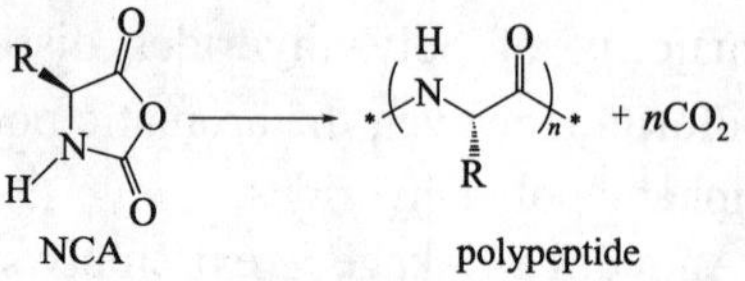

Scheme 5-8. Polymerization of α-animo acid-*N*-carboxyanhydrides (NCAs).

derived from tyrosine dipeptide as monomeric starting material (Scheme 5-9). Pseudo-poly(amino acids) are characterized by the presence of nonamide bonds such as ether, ester, urethane, or carbonate in their backbone structure. The development of pseudo-poly(amino acids) represents an attempt to use naturally occurring amino acids as monomeric building blocks without creating conventional poly(amino acids).

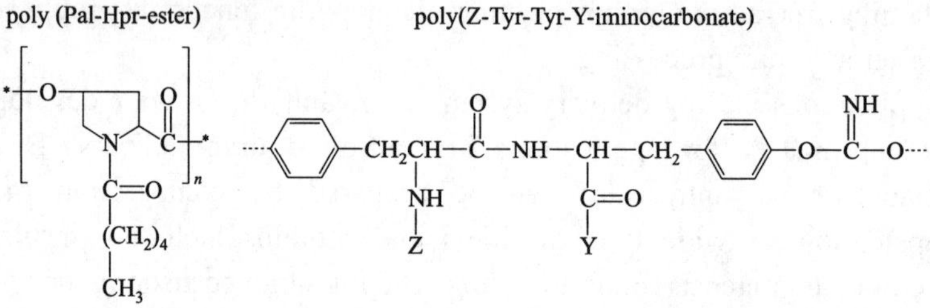

Scheme 5-9. The structures of poly(*N*-acylhydroxyproline esters) and a homologous series of tyrosine-derived polymers.

(2) Typical properties   Poly(amino acids) are generally hydrophilic and biodegradable, showing low systemic toxicity. Their degradation rates are dependent upon hydrophilicity of the amino acids. For example, copolymer of glutamic acid and ethylglutamate containing 13 mol % glutamic acid was reported to remain intact for more than 79 days, while the 40% copolymer disintegrated in 7 days.

Most poly(amino acids) are highly insoluble and nonprocessible due to strong interchain hydrogen bonds, though they have a pronounced tendency to swell in aqueous media. Furthermore, polymers containing three or more amino acids have the risk of antigenicity. Because of these limitations, only a few of poly(amino acids), usually derivates of poly(glutamic acid) carrying various pendant chains at the γ–carboxylic acid group, have been investigated as implant materials. So far, there are still no drug with poly(amino acids) approved for clinical use in the United States.

In "pseudo"-poly(amino acids), half on the amide bonds are replaced by other linkages (such as carbonate, ester or iminocarbonate bonds) that have a much lower tendency to form interchain hydrogen bonds. It endows the polymer with an increased solubility in common organic solvents, reduced water uptake and swelling and generally, a loss of crystallinity, which results in an improvement of the processing behavior.

(3) Applications in drug delivery system   Poly(amino acids) are used as drug delivery carriers since the amino acid side chains offer sites for the attachment of

drugs[13]. The poly(amino acids)-drug combinations investigated include poly(L-lysine) with methotrexate and pepstatin, and poly(glutamic acid) with adriamycin, a widely used chemotherapeutic agent.

Random copolymers of the α-amino acids *N*-(3-hydro-xypropyl)-L-glutamine and L-leucine were synthesized and used as carriers for naltrexone, as shown in Figure 5-2. Naltrexone was covalently bound through the 3-phenolic or the 14-tertiary hydroxyls to the polymer hydroxyl side chains via a carbonate bond. Naltrexone was released from the polymer in a relatively constant way for 30 days, in both in vitro and in vivo experiments in rats.

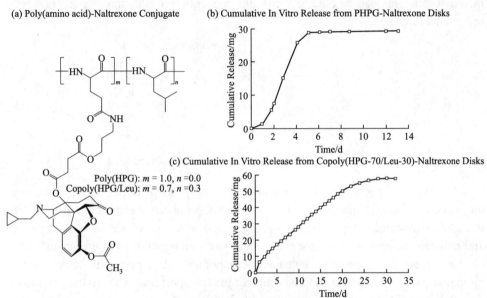

Figure 5-2. Schematic structure of poly(α-amino acid)-Naltrexone conjugate and their in vitro release curves[15].

As for the pseudo-poly(amino acids), no clinical tests have far been conducted, since only a few of them are available presently. But there are active investigations carried out in some laboratories for their medical applications ranging from biodegradable bone nails to implantable adjuvants [1].

5.3.5 Polyphosphazenes

(1) Polymer description   Polyphosphazenes are a kind of unusual polymers, with inorganic backbone consisting of nitrogen-phosphorus bonds (N=P). The general structural formula of polyphosphazenes is shown as below, where the molecules contain two organic or organometallic side groups attached to each phosphorus atom. More than 700 different polyphosphazenes are known, with different side groups (R) and different molecular architectures.

Generally structural formula of polyphosphazenes:

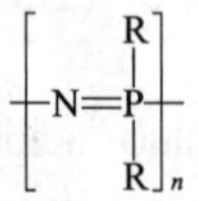

$$\left[\begin{array}{c} R \\ | \\ N{=}P \\ | \\ R \end{array} \right]_n$$

The polymers are most commonly synthesized by a substitution reaction of the reactive poly(dichlorophosphazene) with a wide range of reactive nucleophiles such as amines, alkoxides, and organometallic molecules (Scheme 5-10). Polymers containing mixed substituents can be obtained from the sequential or simultaneous reaction with several nucleophiles.

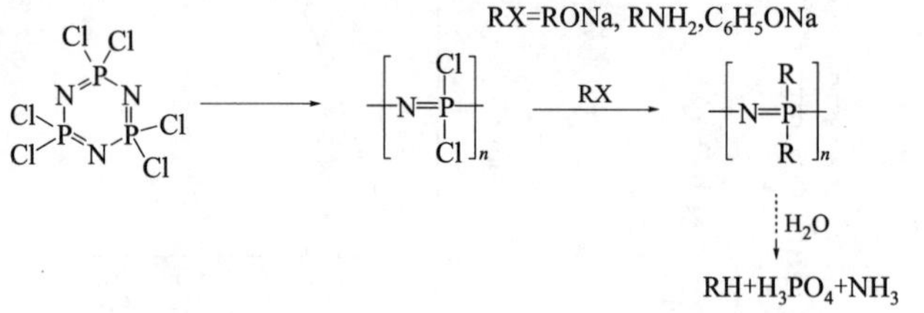

Scheme 5-10. Synthesis and hydrolysis of polyphospazenes.

(2) Typical properties   The uniqueness of polyphosphazenes stems from their inorganic backbone, which is very flexible. Polyphosphazenes exhibit rather low glass transition temperature, high thermal stability, good water resistance, solvent resistance and radiation resistance. Also, the side groups exert an equal or even greater influence on the properties, especially on the hydrophobicity, hydrophilicity, color, useful biological properties such as bioerodibility, or ion transport properties to the polymers.

Polyphosphazenes have been claimed to be biocompatible and biodegradable. The degradation of polyphosphazenes occurrs mainly on their side groups, and the backbone can be hydrolyzed to phosphate and ammonia. It is feasible to control the hydrolysis of poly phosphazens over hours, days, months, or years by controlling the species of side groups.

(3) Applications in drug delivery system   Several types of poly phospha-zenes have been used as matrix carriers for drugs or as a hydrolyzable polymeric drug, where various drugs, peptide or other biological compounds can be covalently bound to the polymer backbone and later released from the polymer via hydrolysis[16]. For example, amino acid ester-substituted polyphosphazenes have been used for controlled release of the covalently bonded anti-inflammatory agent naproxen. Steroids having a hydroxyl group were also bound to the polymer chain through the hydroxyl group. The rates of degradation and release can be controlled by appropriate selection of amino acid side chain groups. The hydrolysis half-lives vary from weeks to months depending on the structure of the amino acid ester.

Another novel use of polyphosphazenes is in the area of vaccine design where these materials were used as immunological adjuvants [17].

◆ 本章中文导读 ◆

生物降解性高分子材料在医药领域已被用作可降解血管支架、骨钉、手术缝线和各种新型给药系统载体材料等。生物降解指通过增溶、水解或生物体中的酶以及其他生物活性物质作用使材料转化成一些较小的复杂的中间产物或终产物的过程。生物降解的范围很广，包括发生在体内的各种类型的降解，无论它是水解还是代谢过程。生物降解性给药系统的降解方式是影响药物释放的重要因素之一。降解方式有两种：表面和本体降解，又称非均相和均相降解。药物随着本体降解或降解之前从聚合物基质中的释放主要以简单扩散方式进行；药物从进行表面降解的聚合物中的释放则取决于药物扩散和基质降解二方面的因素。对于共价结合到聚合物链上的药物分子，药物的释放主要取决于该共价键的降解，而与聚合物降解方式无关。最理想的生物降解性给药系统载体材料是在药物释放和聚合物降解后不留下残余聚合物。本章主要介绍在药剂研究中常用的生物降解性高分子材料。

（1）聚丙交酯、丙交酯–乙交酯共聚物 [poly(lactic acid), poly(lactic-co-glycolic acid) copolymer]　聚丙交酯、丙交酯–乙交酯共聚物是一类应用广泛的生物降解性合成高分子聚酯，其降解是由主链上不稳定的脂肪族酯键水解引起，已被美国 FDA 批准作为微球、微囊、植入剂等剂型的药用辅料。高分子量的聚丙交酯、丙交酯–乙交酯共聚物可由乙交酯和丙交酯通过开环、加聚得到。聚乙交酯具有高度结晶性和生物降解性，不溶于绝大多数有机溶剂。因为丙交酯有 3 种异构体，分别聚合可得到聚（D-丙交酯）、聚（L-丙交酯）和无定形的聚（DL-丙交酯）。聚丙交酯结晶性比聚乙交酯差，可溶于卤代烃、乙酸乙酯、四氢呋喃、二氧杂环己烷等有机溶剂。聚（L-丙交酯）和聚（DL-丙交酯）最常见并得到广泛应用。丙交酯–乙交酯共聚物比其均聚物的结晶性要小，其性能高度可调且变化范围大，可通过改变以下四个关键参数获得：单体立体化学、单体投料比、高分子链的结构和分子量。聚丙交酯、丙交酯–乙交酯共聚物的降解是由主链上不稳定的脂肪族酯键水解引起，水解速率取决于聚合物的分子量、结晶度、样品形状和水解的理化环境。

（2）聚己酸内酯 [poly(ε-caprolactone), PCL]　聚己酸内酯是一种半结晶性生物可降解高分子，可做为微球、植入剂等剂型的药用辅料。聚己酸内酯的重复结构单元由 5 个非极性亚甲基和 1 个极性酯基组成，其机械性能与聚烯烃相似，同时又具有生物降解性，与其他许多聚合物具有罕见的相容性质。高分子量的聚己酸内酯均聚物和共聚物可通过开环、加聚制得。由于分子中脂肪族酯键易被水解，聚己酸内酯及其共聚物都可生物降解。由于聚己酸内酯具有烃类结构特征和结晶性，聚己酸内酯的生物降解要比聚（α-羟基酸）如聚丙交酯慢得多。聚己酸内酯在降解过程中酶的作用很小，引起其降解的一个主要因素是羟基自由基。此外，一些细菌，酵母和真菌均可在一定程度上降解聚己酸内酯。

（3）聚 β-羟基丁酸酯［poly(β-hydroxybutyrate), PHB］ 聚 β-羟基丁酸酯是一种硬而脆的生物降解高分子，目前主要采用微生物发酵法制备，兼有天然可降解材料和人工合成可降解材料的特点。聚 β-羟基丁酸酯具有高度结晶性和热塑性，降解机理为酶解。降解产物 3-羟基丁酸为人体内源性成分，与人体有良好相容性。3-羟基丁酸酯/羟基戊酸酯共聚物近于无定形，适于制备整体溶蚀的骨架片剂。同其他天然可降解材料相比，聚 β-羟基丁酸酯具有生物相容性、压电性、光学活性、无毒性、无刺激性、不易引起受体的免疫反应，又有人工合成可降解材料所具有的机械强度、拉伸度以及很高的耐磨性，且化学性质稳定。这些性质使其成为一种新的组织工程用支架材料，并在药物缓释方面得到广泛的应用。

（4）聚原酸酯［poly(orthoesters), POE］ 聚原酸酯是一种通过原酸酯与多元醇类缩合形成原酸酯键制得的生物可降解高分子材料。已知的聚原酸酯为疏水性高分子，体内的溶蚀仅发生在高分子–水的界面，是一种表面溶蚀。自 20 世纪 70 年代以来，已开发了 4 代聚原酸酯用作药物输送的生物溶蚀性载体。这 4 代聚原酸酯分别表示为聚原酸酯Ⅰ、Ⅱ、Ⅲ和Ⅳ（POE Ⅰ、Ⅱ、Ⅲ和Ⅳ）。聚原酸酯Ⅰ是由无水 2,2-二乙氧基四氢呋喃与二元醇脱去乙醇，缩聚而得，已用于治疗烧伤，纳曲酮、避孕药物类固醇和吲哚美辛的给药系统，以及整形外科等。聚原酸酯Ⅱ可采用二乙烯酮缩二甲醇与多元醇加成反应合成得到，已应用于 5–氟尿嘧啶和纳曲酮给药系统，及避孕药左旋甲炔诺酮植入剂的载体。聚原酸酯Ⅲ可通过原酸酯单体和三元醇单体之间的酯交换反应缩聚制备。其作为药物载体的突出优点是固体药物能直接通过机械方法与其混合均匀，不用加热，也无需溶剂协助，操作简便。可用作辅助治疗青光眼、严重烧伤脓毒症、治疗牙周病，还可应用于兽药。聚原酸酯Ⅳ主链（POE$_x$LA$_y$）上含有乳酸单元，是一类可精密控制原酸酯键的降解速率的新一代高分子，具有黏性，可注射，主要为表面溶蚀。与其他聚原酸酯相比，聚原酸酯Ⅳ在辐射灭菌（包括 β、γ 射线）处理后，分子量和化学结构都没有改变。

（5）聚磷酸酯［poly(phosphate esters)］ 聚磷酸酯为重复单元为磷酸酯基的一类高分子。在生理条件下，聚磷酸酯通过磷酸酯键的水解和可能的酶消化而降解。由于其生物相容性以及与核苷酸等生物大分子的类似性，聚磷酸酯在生物医药方面得到广泛的应用。疏水性聚磷酸酯可以作为小分子药物、蛋白质、DNA 质粒的载体和组织工程支架。聚磷酸酯主链上的五价磷原子可以通过 P—O 键或 P—N 键进行官能化修饰，从而得到具有不同物理化学性质的聚合物。以含 P—H 键的聚亚磷酸酯为反应物，可制备各种水溶性聚磷酸酯。聚磷酸酯主链具有可以降解的磷酸二酯键，被广泛应用于药物缓释、基因传递以及组织工程等领域。

（6）聚酸酐 (polyanhydrides) 聚酸酐是重复单元通过酸酐键连接的生物降解性高分子材料。聚酸酐可采用熔融缩聚、开环聚合、界面缩聚等方法和使用脱水偶合剂来制备，平均分子量一般为 5000～300000，分子量分布指数为 2～15。因其结构单元特点可以分为脂肪族聚酸酐、不饱和聚酸酐、芳香族聚酸酐、脂肪族–芳香族聚酸酐、氨基酸基聚酸酐等。聚酸酐具有如下优点：成本低廉，合成所用单体为二元羧酸；一步合成，无需纯化；结构明确，分子量可控，聚合物的水解速率可以预期；作为载体，可在一定时间内，使药物以一定的速率释放；易于加工，可低温注塑和挤出成型；水解产物二元酸可在几周或几个月内从体内完全消除；采用 γ 射线辐射灭菌，对聚合物性质影响不大。聚酸酐的降解由水解引起，由于酸酐键易于水解，聚酸酐会快速降解为二元酸低聚物和二元羧酸单体。由于降解快，聚酸酐主要应用于控制药物短期释放。聚酸酐用作给药系统的载体，制备双氯乙基亚硝脲（BCNU）植入剂（Gliadel®），已用于临床治疗脑瘤；制备硫酸庆大霉素的植入剂（Septacin™），用于治疗骨髓炎。

（7）聚氨基酸［poly(amino acids)］ 聚氨基酸可分为两类：一类是氨基酸的天然聚合物，如蛋白质、多肽激素、酶及活性肽等；一类是人工合成聚合物，包括天然活性肽及其类似物、聚赖氨酸、聚精氨酸、聚谷氨酸等。对生物体无毒、无副作用、无免疫源性，具有良好的生物相容性，并可通过体内的水解或酶解反应最终降解为小分子的氨基酸，容易被机体吸收和代谢。其所带官能团的侧链，能直接键合药物，也能用贮存或基体方式与药物结合，并且通过改变侧链的亲疏水性、荷电性和酸碱性可调节药物的扩散速率与自身的生物降解性。因此聚氨基酸作为一类较好的药物控制释放载体，在药物控制释放领域得到了大量的研究。

（8）聚磷腈（polyphosphazenes） 聚磷腈是一类具有由 N、P 原子交替通过单、双键交替连接的无机主链的聚合物，通过侧链衍生化引入性能各异的有机基团可以得到理化性质变化范围很广的高分子材料。聚磷腈的生物相容性好，具有生物降解性，一般来说，没有毒性。基于侧基的类型，可将生物降解性聚磷腈分为两类：胺取代生成物——胺化聚磷腈；活化醇取代物——烷氧基聚磷腈。胺化聚磷腈为研究最多也是最大的一类生物降解性聚磷腈。研究表明，含有氟代烷氧基的聚磷腈组织反应性很小，芳氧基聚磷腈很有希望用作惰性生物材料。聚磷腈具有很强的抗菌活性。未发现聚磷腈有诱变性。聚磷腈用于给药系统主要有两种方式：①将药物分子轭合在高分子主链上，属于高分子前药。如类固醇的钠盐与聚二氯磷腈反应键合到聚磷腈分子上，一些局麻药物如普鲁卡因、苯唑卡因和氯普鲁卡因通过氨基与聚磷腈分子链相连。具有生物活性的胺也可通过生成希夫碱而间接连接到聚磷腈上。用相似的方法也可将酶如葡萄糖磷酸酯脱氢酶，胰岛素固定在聚磷腈分子上。②用作骨架材料，药物分子分散在其中。含有咪唑和甲基苯氧侧基的聚磷腈可作为黄体酮和牛血清白蛋白给药系统的骨架材料，聚磷腈氨基酸衍生物可用作抗癌药物如美法仑的载体材料，甘氨酸乙酯聚磷腈、苯丙氨酸乙酯聚磷腈及其共混物可用作抗癌药物丝裂霉素 C 的载体。

References

[1] Comb A J, Kumar N, Sheskin T, Bentolila A, Slager J, Teomin D, Biodegradable Polymers as Drug Carrier Systems, // S. Dumitriu, Editor, Polymeric Biomaterials. CRC Press, 2001: 91.

[2] Kissel T, Brich Z, Bantle S, Lancranjan I, Nimmerfall F, Vit P. Parenteral Depot-Systems on the Basis of Biodegradable Polyesters. Journal of Controlled Release, 1991, 16(1–2): 27–41.

[3] Vert M, Li S, Garreau H. More About the Degradation of La/Ga-Derived Matrices in Aqueous Media. Journal of Controlled Release, 1991, 16(1–2): 15–26.

[4] Jeong B, Bae Y H, Lee D S, Kim S W. Biodegradable Block Copolymers as Injectable Drug-Delivery Systems. Nature, 1997, 388(6645): 860–2.

[5] Vukelja S J, Anthony S P, Arseneau J C, Berman B S, Cunningham C C, Nemunaitis J J, Samlowski W E, Fowers K D. Phase 1 Study of Escalating-Dose Oncogel (Regel/Paclitaxel) Depot Injection, a Controlled-Release Formulation of Paclitaxel, for Local Management of Superficial Solid Tumor Lesions. Anticancer Drugs, 2007, 18(3): 283–9.

[6] DuVall G A, Tarabar D, Seidel R H, Elstad N L, Fowers K D. Phase 2: A Dose-Escalation Study of Oncogel (Regel/Paclitaxel), a Controlled-Release Formulation of Paclitaxel, as Adjunctive Local Therapy to External-Beam Radiation in Patients with Inoperable Esophageal Cancer. Anticancer Drugs, 2009, 20(2): 89–95.

[7] Darney P D, Monroe S E, Klaisle C M, Alvarado A. Clinical Evaluation of the Capronor Contraceptive Implant: Preliminary Report. American Journal of Obstetrics & Gynecology, 1989, 160(5): 1292–1295.

[8] Freier T, Kunze C, Nischan C, Kramer S, Sternberg K, Sass M, Hopt U T, Schmitz K P. In Vitro and in Vivo Degradation Studies for Development of a Biodegradable Patch Based on Poly(3-Hydroxybutyrate). Biomaterials, 2002, 23(13): 2649–57.

[9] Scott G E, Degradable Polymers: Principles and Applications. 2nd edition ed: Springer, 2003: 338.

[10] Heller J, Barr J, Ng S Y, Abdellauoi K S, Gurny R. Poly(Ortho Esters): Synthesis, Characterization, Properties and Uses. Advanced Drug Delivery Reviews, 2002, 54(7): 1015–1039.

[11] K.W.Leong, Controlled Drug Delivery: Challenges and Strategies, ed. K.Park: ACS, 1997.

[12] Dahiyat B I, Richards M, Leong K W. Controlled Release from Poly(Phosphoester) Matrices. Journal of Controlled Release, 1995, 33(1): 13–21.

[13] Kohn J, Abramson S, Langer R, Bioresorbable and Bioerodible Materials // B. Ratner, et al., Editors, Biomaterials Science: An Introduction to Materials in Medicine. Academic Press, 2004.

[14] Kohn J and Langer R. Polymerization Reactions Involving the Side Chains Of .Alpha.-L-Amino Acids. Journal of the American Chemical Society, 1987, 109(3): 817–820.

[15] Negishi N, Bennett D B, Cho C S, Jeong S Y, Van Heeswijk W A, Feijen J, Kim S W. Coupling of Naltrexone to Biodegradable Poly(Alpha-Amino Acids). Pharmaceutical Research, 1987, 4(4): 305–10.

[16] Teasdale I and Bruggemann O. Polyphosphazenes: Multifunctional, Biodegradable Vehicles for Drug and Gene Delivery. Polymers, 2013, 5(1): 161–187.

[17] Eng N F, Garlapati S, Gerdts V, Potter A, Babiuk L A, Mutwiri G K. The Potential of Polyphosphazenes for Delivery of Vaccine Antigens and Immunotherapeutic Agents. Current Drug Delivery, 2010, 7(1): 13–20.

Chapter 6.

Advanced Applications of Functional Polymer in Drug Delivery

功能高分子材料在药物输送中的应用进展

6.1 Hydrogels for pharmaceutical application

6.1.1 Introduction

Hydrogels, as shown in Figure 6-1 are a three-dimensional network of hydrophilic polymers held together by association bonds such as covalent bonds，and weaker cohesive forces，such as hydrogen and ionic bonds and intermolecular hydrophobic association. These networks are able to retain a large quantity of water within their structure without dissolving. Therefore, hydrogels are mostly water by weight while they behave like solids.

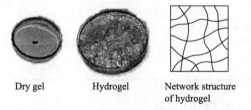

Dry gel   Hydrogel   Network structure
                                   of hydrogel

Figure 6-1. Typical hydrogels and their network structure.

Based on the crosslinking method, hydrogels are basically classified into two groups: the chemical crosslinking hydrogels and the physical crosslinking hydrogels. In the former case, polymer network results from covalent bonds to form insoluble gels. On the other hand, the physical method introduces physical crosslinks between polymer chains through intermolecular force such as hydrogen bonds, van der Waals force, hydrophobic association and so on.

The research of hydrogel as an ideal biocompatible material was pioneered by

Wichterle and Lim, who developed the first synthetic hydrogel and the subsequent application as therapeutic soft contact lenses. Since then the research for hydrogels increased year by year. Table 6-1 gives several examples of physical hydrogels formed by pharmaceutical polymers as mentioned previously.

Table 6-1. Hydrogels examples from several common pharmaceutical polymers.

Polymer example	Hydrogel formation	Cross-linking mechanism	Schematic picture
PVA	Aqueous solutions containing 10%~15% (wt) PVA produce hydrogels after freezing and thawing cycles.	Microcrystalline formed by hydrogen bonds	Microcrystalline Region
Gelatin	Gelatin is dissolved in hot water. The gelatin sol transforms gel when temperature decreases less than 35 °C.	Hydrogen bonds	Cool / Heat
Poloxamer	Solutions of P407 at concentrations of 20% show in situ thermoreversible gelation behavior.	Hydrophobic interaction	Hydrophobic domain
Alginate	Alginate gels usually produced by dripping Ca^{2+} solution into an alginate bath.	Ionical crosslinking	Ca^{2+}

6.1.2 Preparation of hydrogels [1]

Hydrogels are prepared by various methods. Typical methods of preparing hydrogels are irradiation, chemical reactions and physical association. The radiation method utilizes electron beams, gamma rays, X-rays, or ultraviolet light to excite polymer chains to produce a crosslinking point. Chemical crosslinking requires a di- or trifunctional crosslinking agent and polymers with reactive functional groups in the side chain or the chain ends. Another chemical crosslinking method is a simultaneous copolymerization-crosslinking reaction between one or more monomers using polymerizable crosslinking agent. Physical crosslink association introduces physical crosslinks between polymer chains through intermolecular force.

6.1.3 Properties of hydrogels

Hydrogels exhibit superior chemical and physical properties depending on their structures and compositions, which makes them charming as biomedical materials. For example, the low interfacial tension between the hydrogel surface and the aqueous solution can minimize protein adsorption and cell adhesion. The elastic nature of the hydrated hydrogels when used as implants can minimize irritation to surrounding tissue. These characters endow hydrogels with good biocompatibility. Furthermore, the swelling behavior, permeability and stimuli-responsibility of hydrogels will be discussed in detail below.

(1) Swelling behavior   Hydrogels swell distinctly in water, which is driven by the affinity between hydrophilic polymer network and water. The polymer chains of hydrogels interact with the solvent molecule (water) and tend to expand to the fully solvated state. On the other hand, the crosslink structure works as the retractive force to pull back the polymer chain inside. This retractive force is described by the Flory rubber elasticity theory. The counterbalance of the expanding and retracting force attains to equilibrium in a particular solvent at particular temperature.

To describe the swelling behavior of hydrogels, their swelling ratio or water content is currently used in most cases. The swelling ratio is expressed by the ratio of the weight of swollen sample over that of the dry sample:

$$\text{Swelling ratio} = \frac{\text{weight of swollen gel}}{\text{weight of dry gel}}$$

The water content of a hydrogel is expressed in terms of percentage of water by weight:

$$\text{Water content} = \frac{\text{weight of water}}{\text{weight of water} + \text{weight of dry gel}} \times 100$$

For instance, most of hydrogel contact lenses have water content between 38% and 75%. When the water content of the hydrogel is over 90%, the hydrogel is called superabsorbent hydrogel.

The physical behavior of hydrogels is dependent on their equilibrium and dynamic swelling behavior in water, which is a key for the use of hydrogels in biomedical and pharmaceutical applications. The equilibrium swelling ratio influences the solute diffusion coefficient, surface wettability and mobility, and optical and mechanical properties of hydrogels.

(2) Permeability   The permeability of target molecules is important for medical application of hydrogels. For instance, oxygen permeation for contact lens, nutrient and immunological biosubstance transport for immunoisolation and releasing drugs and proteins for drug delivery systems are core characteristics for each application.

(3) Stimuli-responsibility [2]   Some polymers undergo strong conformational changes when only small changes occur in the environment, such as temperature, pH, and ionic strength. When these stimulus-responsive polymers are cross-linked to form a gel, it may exhibit swelling behavior dependent on the external environment and there usually exists a critical point at which the transition occurs. These stimuli-responsive hydrogels are also called smart hydrogel. The mechanism causing the network structural changes can be entirely reversible in nature. Figure 6-2 schematically shows three ways that smart hydrogels are stimulated to release drugs. The corresponding examples are illustrated below in detail.

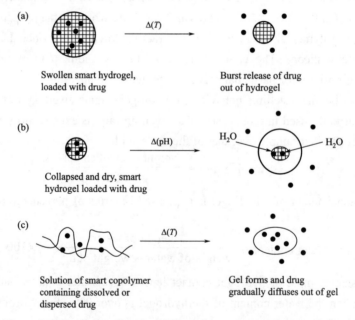

Figure 6-2. Three ways that smart hydrogels are stimulated to release drugs.

One example of smart hydrogels that can reversibly respond to temperature changes is based on N-isopropylacrylamide, as shown in Figure 6-2(a). The hydrogel shrinks abruptly when heated just above 32℃. Here, the collapse of hydrogel occurs as a result of a phase transition of poly(N-isopropylacrylamide) which is soluble in water below its lower critical solution temperature (LCST) of 32℃ but becomes insoluble when the temperature is increased above this temperature. Such materials can deliver biological molecules, where the drug is released accompanying the shrinking of gel triggered by temperature changes.

PH-sensitive hydrogels are another class of environmentally sensitive gels. These hydrogels are swoolen ionic networks containing either acidic or basic pendant groups. In aqueous media of appropriate pH and ionic strength, the pendant groups can ionize developing fixed charges on the gel. As a result, the mesh size of the polymeric networks can change significantly with small pH changes, which will leads to drug release [Figure 6-2(b)]. The most commonly studied ionic polymers include poly(acrylamide) (PAAm), poly(acrylic acid) (PAA), alginate, chitosan and so on.

The triblock copolymers of PEO-PPO-PEO, known as poloxamer, are of more interest having a pronounced thermal gelation capability [Figure 6-2(c)]. Some grades of poloxamer exhibit sol-gel transitions at body temperature in solutions at concentration above 16 wt% and thus may be used for injectable drug delivery system.

6.1.4 Pharmaceutical applications of hydrogels

Hydrogels are attractive for a variety of pharmaceutical applications[3] because of their good tissue compatibility, easy manipulation under swelling condition and solute permeability. Especially, their hydrophilicities can impart desirable release characteristics to controlled and sustained release formulations of drugs and proteins. And hydrogels hold tremendous promise as protein delivery system since the hydrogels show good nondenaturing effects on the incorporated protein.

Generally, there are two methods for loading drugs into hydrogels. Firstly, a hydrogel monomer is mixed with drug, initiator and crosslinker and is polymerized to entrap the drug within the matrix. Secondly, a preformed hydrogel (in most cases lyophilized) is allowed to swell to equilibrium in a suitable drug solution. Nevertheless, pharmaceutical hydrogel systems include equilibrium-swollen hydrogels and swelling-controlled ones. In swelling-controlled release system, the bioactive agents are dispersed into the polymer to form nonporous films, disks, or spheres. When contact with aqueous medium, polymer will be swollen resulting in a distinct interface corresponding to the water penetration. The release of these drugs from the hydrogel delivery system involves absorption of water into the polymer matrix and subsequent diffusion of the drugs outward through the swollen gel, which can be determined by Fick's Law. And the macromolecular relaxations of the polymer influence the diffusion mechanism of the drug through the gel. Overall, factors affecting the drug release from hydrogels include the drug loading method, the local partition of drugs, the overall hydrophilic/hydrophobic balance, the osmotic effect of dissolved drugs, and the polymer chain elasticity. The hydrogel matrix selected for a specific drug carrier should be tailored considering the aforementioned effects as well as the physical properties of drugs and release kinetics.

Some typical examples of hydrogels in pharmacetical applications are introduced herein.

Poly(vinyl alcohol) (PVA) is a hydrophilic polymer receiving much attentions as drug delivery carrier. Two methods exist for the preparation of PVA gels. Linear PVA chains are usually cross-linked using glyoxal or glutaraldehyde to produce the chemically crosslinked PVA hydrogel. Physically crosslinked PVA gels have been prepared by a repeating freeze-thawing process and studied as protein-releasing matrices. This method allows for the formation of an "ultrapure" network without the use of toxic cross-linking agents. By incorporating bovine serum albumin (BSA) as a model protein into the PVA gel, BSA release profiles demonstrated diffusion controlled release and adjusting the number of freeze-thawing cycles resulted in no significant difference in release rate[4]. The initial release of the drug was attributed to diffusion of drug through water-filled pores near the surface of the polymer matrix.

Alginate is one of the most popular natural hydrogel matrices for drug release. Alginate hydrogels are usually formed via ionic interactions between carboxylic acids and divalent cations such as Ca^{2+}, Mg^{2+}, and Ba^{2+}. Ionically crosslinked alginate hydrogels have been used to incorporate several different proteins for controlled release applications[5] including TGF-β1, basic fibroblast growth factor (bFGF), tumor necrosis factor receptor, epidermal growth factor (EGF), and urogastrone. Most of these proteins are incorporated into alginate hydrogels via ionic bonding to the polymer, but sometimes the bioactivity of incorporated proteins is reduced by such ionic interaction. The addition of poly (acrylic acid) to the alginate hydrogel was shown to prevent the inactivation of proteins by alginate.

In addition, stimuli-responsive hydrogels, which exhibit the rapid changes in swelling behavior and pore structure in response to small changes in pH or temperature, are promising as carriers for bioactive agents, including peptides and proteins. And these favorable characteristics lend these materials to serve as self-regulated, pulsatile drug delivery system [6]. For example, a glucose-sensitive insulin releasing system for diabetes therapy was developed using pH-responsive polymer, poly[(*N,N*-dimethylamino) ethyl methacrylate-*co*-ethylacrylamide] [7]. The polymer was mixed and compressed with glucose oxidase, bovine serum albumin, and insulin, as shown in Figure 6-3. When the matrix was exposed to glucose, it was oxidized to form gluconic acid. Then,

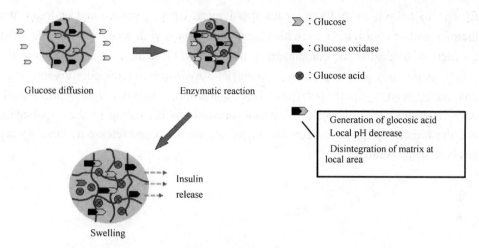

Figure 6-3. Schematic representation of a glucose-controlled insulin release using poly(DMAEMA-*co*-EAAm).

insulin was released as the hydration state was improved by a decrease in the pH.

In the range of smart polymer hydrogels, thermogelling copolymers are included with unique character, which exhibit phase change behaviors of sol-to-gel-to-sol, sol-to-gel or gel-to-sol transition upon an increase in temperature (Figure 6-4)[8]. The formation of gels takes place via physical crosslinking between the copolymers. The phase transition can be adjusted by changing different parameters, such as composition and molecular weight of the copolymer. The sol-to-gel transition is particularly attractive for applications because the drug can be mixed with the aqueous copolymer solutions at low temperatures and be injected into the body, where the higher body temperature would lead to the formation of a gel depot for the sustained release of the drug via diffusion or erosion or the copolymer gel.

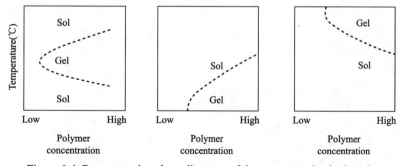

Figure 6-4. Representative phase diagrams of thermoresponsive hydrogels.

Except for poloxamer and some natural polymers, such as gelatin and chitosan, the thermosensitive copolymers have also been incorporated with biocompatible PEG and a variety of biodegradable components such as poly(D,L-lactic acid-*co*-glycolic acid), poly(L-lactic acid), polycarprolactone, poly([R]-3-hydroxybutyrate), poly(organophosphazene), poly(peptide), poly(propylene fumarate), poly(propylene phosphate), polyacetal and poly(ortho ester). Various formulations consisting of the copolymers and therapeutic agents have been developed and the sustained release of these agents has been demonstrated.

◆ **本节中文导读** ◆

药用水凝胶材料：

水凝胶（hydrogel）是亲水性聚合物的三维网状结构，能够吸收大量水分或生理液体而呈现为凝胶状态，一般由均聚物或共聚物通过化学或物理交联形成。由化学交联形成共价键连接的网状结构构成的水凝胶，称之为化学凝胶。通过分子缠结和/或离子键、氢键、疏水作用等二级力构建而成的水凝胶，称为物理凝胶或"可逆"凝胶。

水凝胶具有较高的含水量和"柔软"的质地，因此其与生物组织具有良好的相似性与相容性。水凝胶已广泛用于接触镜片、生物传感器膜、人造器官材料与药物输送系统。在药物输送领域，水凝胶除了可用于小分子药物的控制释放外，还可包封蛋白质、DNA 等生物大分子，由于不存在疏水作用，避免了不稳定生物大分子的失活。交联度是影响水凝胶溶胀的重要因素，从而影响药物的释放速率。近年来受到广泛关注的环境敏感性水凝胶，自身能感知外界环境（如温度、pH 值、光、电、压力等) 微小的变化或刺激，从而产生相应的物理结构和化学性质变化（如凝胶溶胀度的变化、凝胶-溶胶转变等），常被称为智能水凝胶。环境敏感性水凝胶的这种智能性使之在药物的缓控释、蛋白质的分离提纯、活性酶的包埋和人工肌肉等方面有着广阔的应用前景。

6.2 Polymer–based nanomedicine and self–assemblying polymers

6.2.1 Introduction to nanomedicine

Nanomedicine is a subfield of nanotechnology that uses nanomaterials for the diagnosis and treatment of disease[9]. It is well known that when a substance is engineered to be nano-sized (less than 100nm in one dimension), it exhibits unique properties differing greatly from its bulk-sized counterpart. These unique properties have been exploited to create new diagnostics and therapeutics which will be applied in a broad spectrum of diseases such as cancer, cardiovascular and infectious diseases. Nanomedicine could provide new technological advances not only in development of novel drugs, but also in reformulation of already existing drugs to increase their efficacy, improve delivery and lower side effects. Nanomedicine is advanced to target regions of the body that were previously hard to access using traditional drug formulation methods.

In the field of nanomedicine the term nanoparticle is more flexible and includes particles up to 1μm. Nanoparticles can be synthesized in a wide range of shapes and sizes, depending on the molecular basis of the structure, and can be termed soft (organic) or hard (inorganic). Indeed, nanosized structures have been investigated for drug delivery for more than 30 years, such as dendrimers and liposomes. And there are a number of nanomedicines already in clinical use based on these nano-platforms [10]. Besides them, the polymer-based nanocarrier platforms, including polymeric micelles and polymer-drug conjugates, have also proven to be useful in drug delivery carriers [11]. Especially, polymeric micelles are currently recognized as one of the most promising modalities of drug carriers [12]. Polymeric micelles have several advantages, such as a simple preparation, efficient drug loading without chemical modification of the parent drug, tailored drug release and easy functionalizations with moieties that enhance site-specific delivery. Table 6-2 lists the micelle-based nanomedicines that have been approved for clinical use or is undergoing clinical trials.

6.2.2 Micellation of self–assemblying polymers

It is fascinating that block or graft copolymers consisting of incompatible segments would self-assembly in selective solvent or solvent mixture (e.g., good or marginal for one block and poor for the other) to generate nanosized supramolecular

Table 6-2.   Micelle-based nanomedicines that have been approved for clinical use or undergoing clinical trials [13].

Brand name	Composition	Indication	Status
Genexol-PM	Paclitaxel-loaded PEG-PLA micelle	Breast cancer, lung cancer	Approved
NK911	Doxorubicin-loaded PEG-pAsp micelle	Various cancers	Phase 2
NK012	SN-38-loaded PEG-PGlu(SN-38) micelle	Breast cancer	Phase 2
NC-6004	Cisplatin-loaded PEG-PGlu micelle	Various cancers	Phase 1
SP1049C	Doxorubicin-loaded pluronic micelle	Gastric cancer	Phase 3
NK105	Paclitaxel-loaded PEG-PAA micelle	Breast cancer	Phase 3

Notes: PLA, poly(L-lactide); pAsp, poly(L-aspartic acid); PGlu, polyglutamate; PAA, poly(L-aspartate); HPMA, N-(2-hydroxypropyl)-methacrylamide copolymer.

structures [14]. Polymeric micelles are representatives of such supramolecular structures that have attracted intense attention for their potentials in biological applications.

Figure 6-5 shows the self-assemblying behavior of an amphiphilic AB type block copolymer in aqueous media, which typically generates a unique core-shell architecture where the hydrophobic core is segregated from the aqueous exterior by the corona comprised of hydrophilic segments. The micellation of an amphiphilic block copolymer is driven by the interplay of two forces. One is an attractive force, such as hydrophobic interaction, that leads to the association of molecules while the other force, a repulsive one, prevents unlimited growth of the micelles into a macroscopic phase [15]. The association of unimers occurs when their concentration in solution reaches a threshold value known as the critical micellization concentration (CMC). The CMC is therefore defined as the concentration of unimer at a given temperature at which micelles first appear. The CMCs of block copolymer micelles are typically ranging from 10^{-6}mol/L to 10^{-7}mol/L and are significantly lower than CMCs of low-molecular-weight surfactants which range from 10^{-3}mol/L to 10^{-4}mol/L. Generally,

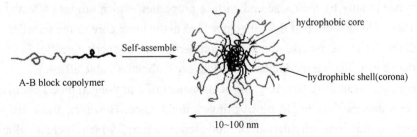

Figure 6-5. Schematic formation of spherical micelle from diblock copolymer.

polymeric micelles are more stable and have a slower rate of dissociation. These properties allow retention of the loaded drugs in polymer micelles for a longer period of time and eventually achieve higher accumulation of a drug at the target site.

A variety of constituent block/graft copolymers can be used for the preparation of polymeric micelles. The hydrophilic polymers with a flexible nature like PEGs are commonly selected as shell-forming segments, which assemble into dense corona to give effective steric stabilization properities. The hydrophobic core is made up of lipid molecules, like poly(propylene oxide), poly(L-amino acid)s, or poly(ester)s. Commonly used poly (L-amino acids) are poly(L-aspartate) and poly(L-glutamate), which can be derivatized at their functional groups. In addition to hydrophobic interaction, the driving force for core segregation also includes electrostatic interaction, metal complexation, and hydrogen bonding[16].

Polyion complex (PIC) micelles are ones generated by the electrostatic interaction between charged block copolymers and oppositely charged macromolecules. The polymer in PIC micelle always contains a nonionic water-soluble segment [e.g., polyethylene glycol (PEG)] and an ionic segment that can be neutralized by oppositely charged polymer chain to form a hydrophobic core, while the core of micelle is stabilized by the nonionic water-soluble shell. This system is potentially useful for the delivery of genes and small interfering RNA (siRNA).

Generally, the structure of polymeric micelles is characterized by their size, size distribution, zeta potential, microstructure, dimension of the core, aggregation number of the polymer chains, and density of the micelles. Size and size distribution of the polymeric micelles can be determined by static and dynamic light scattering (DLS) as well as microscopic techniques.

6.2.3 Biological significance of polymeric micelles

The distribution of drug-loaded polymeric micelles in the body may be determined mainly by their size and surface properties, which are less affected by the properties of loaded drugs if they are embedded in the inner core of the micelles. In this regard, the design of the size and surface properties of polymeric micelles is of crucial importance in achieving modulated drug delivery with remarkable efficacy.

For successful drug targeting, the achievement of a prolonged blood circulation of polymeric nanocarriers might be of primary importance. However, there are several obstacles to the long circulation of polymeric carriers, which include glomerular excretion by the kidney and recognition by the reticuloendothelial system (RES) located in the liver, spleen and lung. The glomerular excretion can be avoided by using polymeric carriers with a larger size than its threshold value (42000~50000 for water-soluble polymers). It is significant that the hydrophilic and flexible coronas give stealth properties to polymeric micelles due to their steric repulsion effect, allowing them to avoid uptake by the RES, which is crucial for achieving long circulation time in blood [12].

The typical biodistribution of polymeric micelles can be exemplified by the results of polymeric micelles composed of PEG-block-poly(D,L-lactide) (PEG-*b*-PDLLA) copolymers labeled with ^{125}I, as reported by K. Kataoka [17]. The PEG-*b*-PDLLA micelles showed a remarkably prolonged blood circulation ($t_{1/2}$ ca. 18h) after intravenous administration, and maintained 25% of the injected dose in the circulation at 24h post-injection. The distribution volume in the central compartment (V_0) and plasma-to-blood ratio of the micelles were calculated to be nearly equivalent to the blood volume and the plasma space value, respectively, suggesting that polymeric micelles might distribute only to the blood compartment and hardly interact with blood cells immediately after their administration.

Moreover, it has been demonstrated that long-circulating polymeric nanocarriers including polymeric micelle can preferentially and effectively accumulate in various types of solid tumors due to the "Enhanced Permeability and Retention (EPR) effect"[18]. EPR effect is explained by the microvascular hyperpermeability to circulating macromolecules and their impaired lymphatic drainage in solid tumors. It has been reported that the vascular pore cut-off sizes of tumors range between 380 and 780 nm for various tumors including mammary and colorectal carcinomas, hepatoma, glioma, and sarcoma [19, 20]. Hence, transvascular transport of polymeric micelles seems to be free due to their relatively small size (i.e., less than 100nm), resulting in an enhanced accumulation in solid tumors. The EPR effect has become a strategic basis for designing polymeric micelles for successful tumor targeted therapy.

6.2.4 Drug release from polymeric micelles

As shown in Figure 6-6, drug can be loaded within polymeric micelles by chemical conjugation or physical entrapment, and the respective drug release processes are dependent on the type of encapsulation. In the chemically conjugated drug, the release occurs by bulk degradation of polymer matrix or surface erosion. Drugs that are physically entrapped may be released from micelles either through diffusion or upon disassociation of the micelle structure, which is influenced by those factors such as the amount of drug loaded, length of the core-forming part of the polymer, and presence and extent of cross-linking. Cross-linking can occur either in the core or throughout the

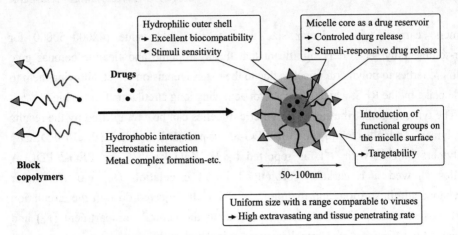

Figure 6-6. Polymeric micelles as intelligent nanocarriers for drug.

shell [21]. Such chemical fixation would increase the stability of the micelles at concentrations even below CMC of the block copolymer.

A desired drug delivery system should release drug with temporal and distribution controls. Temporal control covers the ability to adjust the period of time over which the drug release is supposed to take place or the capability to trigger drug release at a specific time during treatment. Distribution control refers to delivery or release of the drug at a specific site of treatment. Recent advances in synthetic polymer chemistry and biotechnology have allowed the development of polymeric micelles with integrated smart functions, such as environmentally sensitivity and specific tissue target ability, to match aforementioned demands. Tailoring of the polymeric micelles involves various methods [22], such as engineering the block copolymers, cross-linking in the core or shell of the micelles, surface functionalization of the micelles, the addition of auxiliary agents to the micelles and so on.

6.2.5 Examples of polymeric micelles for drug delivery

(1) Delivery of hydrophobic drugs Polymeric micelles formed by amphiphilic block copolymers have been used to solubilize and deliver poorly soluble hydrophobic drugs. BIND-014 (BIND Biosciences) is a polymeric micelle from poly(D,L-lactide) (PLA) and PEG block copolymers, which has a hydrophobic core for the encapsulation of docetaxel (DTXL), and a hydrophilic surface for prolonged circulation. It is also decorated by targeting ligand to target prostate-specific membrane antigen (PSMA) expressing cells [23]. Initial in vitro studies conducted with the PSMA-targeting RNA aptamer A10 as targeting ligand demonstrated a 77-fold increase in cell association of

PSMA-targeted formulations compared to ligand-lacking formulations. In mice bearing human PSMA-positive prostate xenograft tumors, targeted poly(lactic-co-glycolic acid) (PLGA)-based nanoparticles delivered 3.77-fold more chemotherapeutic agent to tumors compared to ligand-lacking control nanoparticles after 24h [24]. In later preclinical studies, optimized BIND-014 treatment caused significant tumor growth inhibition in a mouse xenograft prostate tumor model compared to ligand-lacking controls. In contrast, no difference in anti-tumor effect was observed in PSMA-negative xenograft models. BIND-014 is currently undergoing a phase I clinical trial to determine the safety in patients with advanced or metastatic cancer. Interim data in 3 patients demonstrated that DTXL plasma levels are two orders of magnitude higher when administered as BIND-014 compared to solvent-based DTXL. Full phase I results with BIND-014 in patients with advanced solid tumors revealed an anti-tumor response in 9 out of 28 patients. Phase II studies aimed to evaluate the safety and efficacy of BIND-014 in patients with metastatic castration-resistant prostate cancer or as second-line therapy for patients with lung cancer have recently been initiated [25].

(2) Polymer-metal complex micelles for delivery of platinous drugs   Cisplatin [cis-dichlorodiammineplatinum (II)] (CDDP) is a metal complex antitumor agent widely used for treating many malignancies. However, CDDP exhibits a very short circulation period after systemic injection and its clinical use is limited due to toxic side effects such as acute nephrotoxicity and chronic neurotoxicity. Recently, Kataoka et al. [12] prepared a class of polymeric micelles incorporating CDDP through the polymer-metal complex formation between CDDP and PEG-b-P(Asp) or PEG-block-(glutamic acid) [PEG-b-P(Glu)] copolymers. This micelle formation is based on the ligand substitution reaction of the Pt(II) from chloride (leaving group) to carboxylate in the block copolymers as shown in Figure 6-7. The CDDP-loaded micelles have a diameter of ca. 30 nm with a narrow size distribution and showed a remarkable stability in distilled water. But in physiological saline (0.15mol/L NaCl), the inverse ligand substitution reaction of Pt (II) from the carboxylate to chloride ions occurs, which lead to the slow release of CDDP from micelles, accompanied by the dissociation of the micellar structure with an induction period of ca. 10h. When intravenously injected into tumorbearing mice, CDDP-loaded micelles showed >60% of injected dose in the plasma up to 8 h and significant accumulation in solid tumors (a 20-fold higher concentration than free CDDP). Consequently, the CDDP-loaded micelles exhibited in vivo antitumor activity equivalent to or better than free CDDP

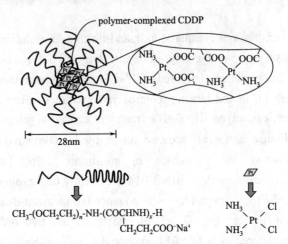

Figure 6-7. Chemical structures of CDDP and PEG-b-P(Glu) copolymers, and schematic illustrations of CDDP-loaded micelles.

and a significantly reduced nephrotoxicity and neurotoxicity, which are expected to be a promising formulation of CDDP for clinical cancer chemotherapy.

(3) Smart polymeric micelles for site-specific drug delivery   There has recently been a strong impetus to the development of polymeric micelles with smart functions, such as targetability to specific tissues and chemical or physical stimuli-sensitivity. Smart polymeric micelles are aimed to increase the selectivity and efficiency of drug delivery to the target cells, leading to a better therapeutic efficacy as well as reduced side effects. Several intracellular signals, such as low pH, glutathion and specific enzymes have been so far used for designing the environmentally sensitive polymeric nanocarriers[26].

◆ **本节中文导读** ◆

纳米制剂与自组装高分子：

纳米颗粒具有尺寸小、比表面积大、表面反应活性高、吸附能力强等特性，在药物筛选、基因转染、疾病诊断、药物输送、检测成像、疾病示踪等方面都有重要作用。将纳米技术应用于药物制剂的研发诞生了纳米制剂。具有精确表面模式的纳米颗粒作为药物载体具有很多优点，能提高难溶性药物的溶解度、实现靶向输送、降低毒副作用等，在缓控释给药、靶向给药、黏膜和局部给药以及基因治疗等领域中显示出特殊的优势。尤其在肿瘤治疗方面，由于肿瘤组织生长快速，其血管壁上存在纳米尺度的高通透性孔状缝隙，抗癌药物的纳米制剂易于穿过这些缝隙到达肿瘤组织内部，即通过肿瘤组织特殊的 EPR 效应实现被动靶向给药。

目前已有多种纳米材料被用作药物载体，根据纳米粒的结构特征，包括：脂质体、树枝状大分子、高分子胶束等。

高分子胶束通常由两亲性高分子通过自组装形成。由两个或两个以上的互不相容的链段或嵌段组成的两亲性高分子（嵌段或接枝共聚物），由于两种链段性质差异大，在水溶液中具有自组装特性。以 AB 型嵌段聚合物为例，其中一个链段为疏水性或非极性的，另一个链段为亲水性或极性的。不同链段的溶解性差异导致胶束化，嵌段高分子在水中组装成纳米尺度的超分子结构－胶束。大多数嵌段共聚物胶束是球形的，由疏水性链段构成相对致密的核和亲水性链段构成外冠。这类高分子纳米胶束可以增溶/负载溶解性差的疏水性药物，其外层的亲水性壳能减少药物与细胞和蛋白之间不必要的相互作用，从而实现药物的安全有效输送。进一步还可以在高分子胶束上接入一些靶向分子和特异分子来增强靶向特异性，达到高效低毒的目的。

应用于药物输送的自组装高分子，亲水性链段通常由水溶性的聚乙二醇构成，疏水性链段中研究最多的是聚环氧丙烷、聚酯和聚（L-氨基酸）。此外，除了疏水性相互作用，通过静电作用使高分子链段缔合也可形成高分子胶束。将带有相反电荷嵌段的两种共聚物混合可形成聚离子复合物（polyion complex, PIC）胶束，如将聚乙二醇-聚 L-赖氨酸（PEG-*b*-PLL）和聚乙二醇-聚天门冬氨酸（PEG-*b*-PAsp）嵌段共聚物配对复合将产生新型的疏水域，可负载药物。

6.3 Polymer–drug conjugates

6.3.1 Introduction

In polymer-drug conjugates, a drug is covalently linked to polymers such as polysaccharides or synthetic polymers. Polymer-drug conjugation is a well known technique useful for improving therapeutic properties of peptides, proteins, small molecules or oligonucleotides. This technology was exploited for the first time in the fifties and sixties in last century and is fast expanding with innovation in the design and production of biotech drugs. Polymer-conjugated drugs generally exhibit prolonged half-life, higher stability, water solubility, lower immunogenicity and antigenicity and often also specific targeting to tissues or cells. There are already several polymer-drug conjugates available in the market or in clinical trial for the treatment of different diseases, as shown in Table 6-3 and Table 6-4.

Table 6-3. Therapeutic products of Polymer-protein and polymer-drug conjugates in the market.

Product	Trade Name	Company	Indication	Approval Year
Polymer-protein conjugates				
Styrene Maleic Anhydride-Neocarzinostatin (SMANCS) (intrahepatic artery)	Zinostatin Stimaler®	Yamanouchi	Hepatocellular carcinoma	1993
PEG-adenosine deaminase (intramuscular)	Adagen®	Enzon	Severe combined immune deficiency syndrome	1990
PEG-L-asparaginase (intravenous or intramuscular)	Oncospar®	Enzon	Acute lymphocytic leukaemia	1994
PEG-interferon α-2b (subcutaneous)	PEG-INTRON®	Schering	Chronic hepatitis C	2000
PEG-interferonα-2a (subcutaneous)	PEGASYS®	Roche	Chronic hepatitis C	2002
PEG-human G-CSF (subcutaneous)	Neulasta®	Amgen	Febrile neutropenia	2002

Continued

Product	Trade Name	Company	Indication	Approval Year
PEG-HGH antagonist (subcutaneous)	Somavert®	Pfizer	Acromegaly	2003
PEG-antiTNF Fab (subcutaneous)	Cimzia®	UCB Pharma	Crohn's disease Arthritis	2008
Polymer-drug conjugate				
Polyglutamic acid-paclitaxel (intravenous)	XYOTAXTM, OPAXIOTM	Cell Therapeutics	NSCLC	Filed EMEA

Table 6-4. Examples of polymer-drug conjugates in clinical development.

Product	Trade name	Company	Indication	Clinical phase
PEGylated-anti VEGFR2 Fab fragments as an angiogenesis inhibitor	CDP 791	UCB Pharma	Non-small cell lung cancer	Phase II
PEG-docetaxel (intravenous)	NKTR-105	Nektar	Solid tumors including hormone-refractory prostate cancer	Phase I
Polyglutamate-camptothecin	CT-2106	Cell therapeutics	Colorectal, lung and ovarian cancer	Phase I
Polyglutamate-pacitaxel	CT-2103,XYOTAX	Cell therapeutics	Cancer,in particular lung, ovarian and es-ophageal cancers	Phase II/ III
PEG-irinotecan (intravenous)	NKTR-102	Nektar	Colorectal, breast, ovarian and cervical cancers	Phase III
PEG-naloxone (oral)	NKTR-118	Nektar	Opioid-induced constipation	Phase III
PEG-camptothecin	PROTHECAN	Enzon	Solid tumors	Phase II
HPMA copolymer platinate (intravenous)	ProLindac®	Access Pharmaceuticals	Ovarian cancer	Phase II
HPMA copolymer–doxorubicin;	PK1; FCE28068	CRC/Pharmacia	Cancer, in particular lung, breast cancers	Phase II
HPMA copolymer–doxorubic in-galactosamine	PK2; FCE28069	CRC/Pharmacia	Hepatocellular carcinoma	Phase I/ II

From a need to progress an industrial development pipeline, Prof. Duncan [11] coined the term "polymer therapeutics" in the 1990s to encompass polymeric drugs, polymer-drug conjugates, polymer-protein conjugates, polymeric micelles to which drug is covalently bound, and those multi-component polyplexes with covalent linkages being developed as non-viral vectors. All these families contain a water-soluble polymer either as an inherently bioactive polymer, or as part of a covalent conjugate. Nowadays, this field witnessed a great development in both the introduction of new and different polymers and the progresses in the chemical strategies of coupling [27].

6.3.2 Design and development of polymer–drug conjugates

(1) Ringsdorf's model   The model for polymer-drug conjugate was proposed by Ringsdorf [28] in 1975. In Ringsdorf's original model (Figure 6-8), a number of drug molecules are bound to a macromolecule through a spacer molecule, which can incorporate a predetermined breaking point to ensure release of the drug at the site of interest. Though the high hydrodynamic volume of the macromolecular carriers offers a passive targeting to solid tumors due to EPR effect, the polymer conjugate can additionally contain moieties (such as antibodies) to target disease related antigens or receptors. In addition, solubilizing groups can be attached to the polymer backbone to modify the bioavailability of the polymer-drug conjugate.

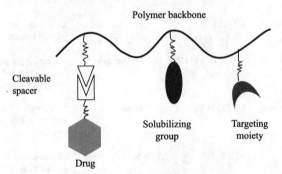

Figure 6-8. Small drug-polymer conjugate model according to Ringsdorf [28].

(2) Basic principles for polymer-drug conjugate design   The rational polymers and conjugation method are two basic principles to build well-defined polymer-drug conjugates.

In general, an ideal polymer for drug conjugation should be characterized by (i) biodegradability or adequate molecular weight that allows elimination from the body to avoid progressive accumulation in vivo; (ii) low polydispersity, to ensure an acceptable homogeneity of the final conjugates; (iii) longer body residence time either to prolong the conjugate action or to allow distribution and accumulation in the desired body compartments; and (iv) for protein conjugation, only one reactive group to avoid crosslinking, whereas for small drug conjugation, many reactive groups to achieve a satisfactory drug loading. Many polymers have been investigated as candidates for the delivery of natural or synthetic drugs as listed below.

① *Synthetic polymers* PEG, *N*-(2-hydroxypropyl)-methacrylamide copolymers (HPMA), poly(acroloylmorpholine) (PAcM), poly(vinylpyrrolidone) (PVP), polyamidoamines, divinylethermaleic anhydride/acid copolymer (DIVEMA), poly(styrene-co-maleic acid/anhydride) (SMA), polyvinylalcohol (PVA);

② *Natural polymer* dextran, pullulan, mannan, dextrin, chitosans, hyaluronic acid, proteins;

③ *Pseudosynthetic polymers:* poly(glutamic acid) (PGA), poly(L-lysine), poly(malic acid), poly(aspartamides), poly((Nhydroxyethyl)-*L*-glutamine) (PHEG).

In addition to Ringsdorf's model, a spectrum of other synthetic polymers with structural and architectural variations, including i) monofunctional linear, ii) polyfunctional linear, iii) starlike, and iv) dendritic architectures are being investigated today, as shown in Figure 6-9.

On the other hand, careful tailoring of polymer–drug linkers is essential to the creation of a polymeric prodrug that is inert during transport but allows drug liberation

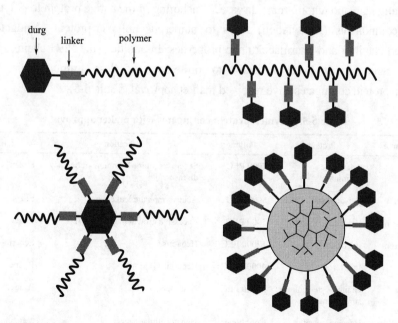

Figure 6-9. Possible structural and architectural types of drug-polymer conjugates.

at an appropriate rate at the site of action. Several methods have been developed primarily based on either hydrolytically unstable bond or enzymatically labile spacers between the drug and the polymer.

Another challenge is to know how the conjugated drug acts and in which form (i.e., whether drug release is essential or the conjugated compound is also active). Usually, a covalent and strategically positioned linkage with the polymer prevents the activity of small drugs.

It is worth noting that though polymer-protein and polymer-drug conjugates share many common features, the biological rationale for their design is a little different. To synthesize polymer-protein conjugate, a semi-telechelic polymer with a single reactive group at one terminal end is required to avoid protein crosslinking during conjugation. The introduction of a linker should not generate toxic or immunogenic by-products and will provide appropriate stability characteristics (dependent on the protein being bound).

6.3.3　Examples for polymer–drug conjugates

(1) Polymer-protein conjugates　Therapeutically relevant proteins such as antibodies, cytokines, growth factors, and enzymes are playing an increasing role in the treatment of viral, malignant, and autoimmune diseases. Anchoring of the native protein to polyethylene glycol components (PEGylation) leads to numerous polymer-protein conjugates with improved stability and pharmacokinetic properties. In addition, the PEG chains mask the protein rendering it more resistant to proteases and less immunogenic. Several polymer-protein conjugates have received market approval (Table 6-5).

Table 6-5. Polymer-protein conjugates with maket approval.

Trade name	Protein	Polymer	Indication	Marketed
Adagen	Adenosine deaminase	5000 PEG	Severe combined immunodeficiency disease	Enzon
Oncaspar	Asparaginase	5000 PEG	Acute lymphatic leukemia	Enzon
Pegvisomant	GH antagonist	5000 PEG	Excessive growth (acromegaly)	Pfizer
PEG-intron	Interferon α2b	12000 PEG	Hepatitis C	Schering-Plough
Pegasys	Interferon α2a	40000 PEG	Hepatitis C	Roche
Neulasta	Granulocyte colony stimulating factor	20000 PEG	Neutropenia	Amgen
SMANCS/lip iodol	Neocarzinostatin	Copolymer of styrene maleic acid	Hepatocellular cancer	Yamanouchi Pharmaceutical Company

In the past few years, either linear PEG chains with a molecular weight between 5000 and 12000 or branched PEG chains are bound to the surface of the protein. In most cases, activated PEG-carboxylic acids, for example, activated with N-hydroxysuccinimide, are bound to the ε-amino groups of lysine residues or the N-terminal amino group, and other chemical modifications with aldehyde, tresylate, or maleimide derivatives of PEG are also used.

(2) Polymer-anti-tumor drug conjugates with cleavable linkers   Conjugation of low molecular-weight anti-tumor drugs to hydrophilic polymers through a cleavable linker provides the opportunity to solubilize poorly water soluble drugs, improve tumour targeting and reduce drug toxicity. Several 'simple' polymer-drug conjugates have now entered Phase I / II clinical trial.

A doxorubicin-(HPMA copolymer) conjugate PK1 was the first polymer-drug conjugate to enter clinical trials [29]. PK1 has a molecular weight of approximately 28 kDa and contains doxorubicin (about 8.5 wt%) linked through its amino sugar to the HPMA copolymer by a tetrapeptide spacer, Gly-Phe-Leu-Gly [Scheme 6-1(a)]. This peptide sequence is cleaved by lysosomal enzymes of tumor cells. A phase I study revealed that the maximum tolerated dose (MTD) was 320 mg $\cdot$ m^{-2} doxorubicin equivalents, which is a fivefold increase relative to the standard dose for doxorubicin.

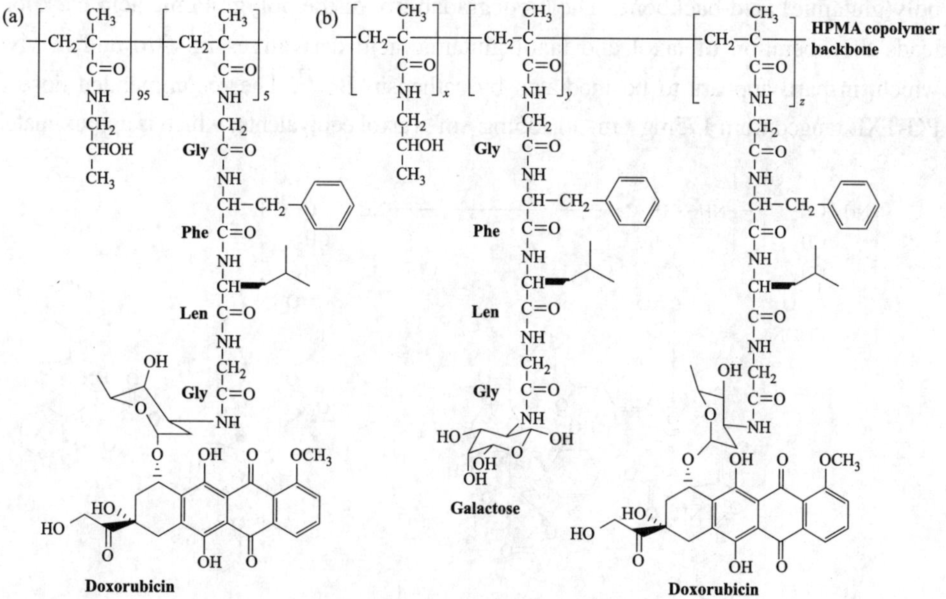

Scheme 6-1. Chemical structure of PK1 (a) and PK2 (b).

No acute cardiotoxicity was observed even at these high doses. The recommended dose for phase II studies was 280mg·m^{-2} every three weeks. Phase II trials in breast, non-small-cell lung and colon cancer were initiated at the end of 1999; an interim report indicated positive responses in a few cases[30].

PK2 is a related compound to PK1, but incorporates an additional targeting ligand, a galactosamine group that was designed to recognize the asialoglycoprotein receptor of liver tumor cells [Scheme 6-1(b)]. In a phase I study, 31 patients with primary or metastatic liver cancer were evaluated. The MTD of PK2 was 160 mg·m^{-2} doxorubicin equivalents which is approximately half the MTD value of PK1, although the molecular weight and the loading ratio are very similar in both conjugates. Dose-limiting toxicity was associated with severe fatigue, neutropenia, and mucositis. A dose of 120mg·m^{-2} doxorubicin equivalents was recommended for phase II studies. Detailed reviews on the clinical studies of polymer-drug conjugates with HPMA copolymer have recently been published by Duncan et al.

PG-TXL (CT-2103), a poly(L-glutamic acid) conjugate of taxol (paclitaxel) (Scheme 6-2), is probably the most successful polymer-drug conjugate to date and is currently undergoing phase III trials in combination with standard chemotherapy against ovarian cancer and non-small-cell lung cancer. PG-TXL has a higher loading ratio about ca. 37 wt% taxol, where the taxol is linked through its 2'-OH group to the poly(glutamic) acid backbone. The biodegradability of the polyglutamic acid backbone leads the liberation of taxol and taxol glutamic acid derivatives in vitro and in vivo, which, in part, appears to be mediated by cathepsin B [31]. The recommended dose of PG-TXL ranged from 175mg·m^{-2} to 235mg·m^{-2} (taxol equivalents) which is approximately

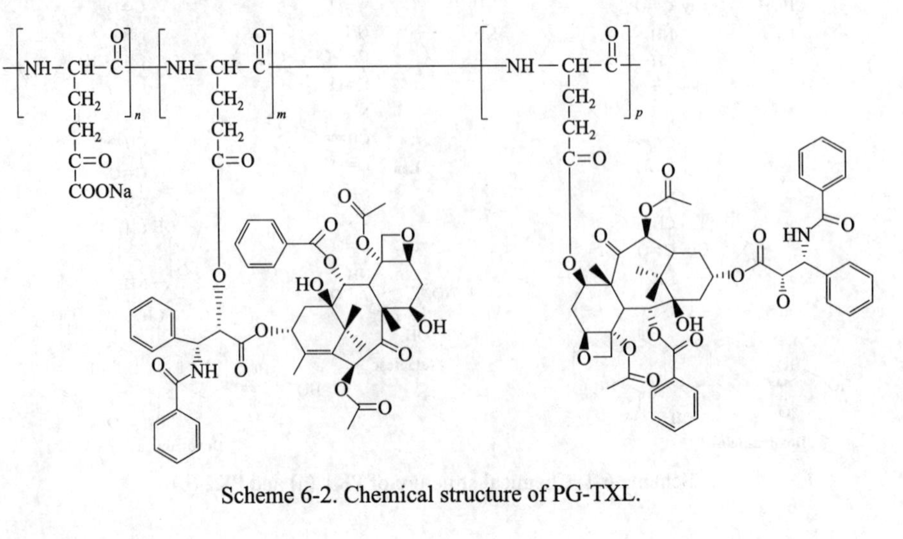

Scheme 6-2. Chemical structure of PG-TXL.

twice as high as for free taxol. Phase I and II studies of various cancers showed promising response rates, even for patients who were resistant to taxane therapy.

Prothecan, a camptothecin conjugate, is the first drug conjugate with polyethylene glycol that has been clinically assessed (Scheme 6-3). Camptothecin was conjugated by the 20-OH with PEG through an ester linker. Here, the esterification of the 20-hydroxy group of camptothecin stabilizes the drug in its active lactone form (closed E ring) which otherwise tends to hydrolyze under physiological conditions and leads to the inactive hydroxycarboxylic acid form. The resulted conjugate is a highly water-soluble formulation of camptothecin due to the use of hydrophilic PEG. Prothecan is currently being assessed in phase II studies for the treatment of gastric and gastroesophageal tumors after a phase I study showed moderate nonhematologic toxicities at its MTD of 200 mg·m^{-2} camptothecin equivalents [32].

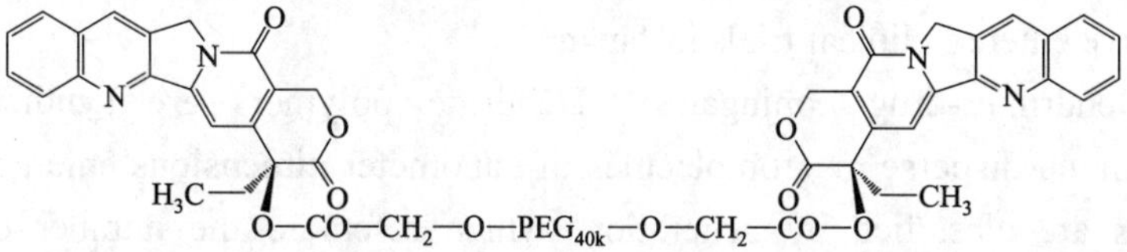

Scheme 6-3. Chemical structure of Prothecan, a camptothecin derivative with PEG.

(3) Block copolymer micelles   Polymeric micelles are generally formed by self-assembly of amphiphilic block copolymer in water, which are more stable than micelles of small surfactant molecules. In traditional micellar formulations, drug was non-covalently entrapped by solubilization. An advanced manner is that the active drug molecules are covalently coupled with the inner block of such nanocarriers, while the terminal functionalities on the outer block (the shell) may incorporate potential targeting properties and control biocompatibility.

For example, Kataoka and co-workers have recently reported the pH-sensitive polymeric micelles for doxorubicin (NK911; 42 nm in diameter),which include a fraction of doxorubicin(about 45%) that is covalently bound to the PEG (M_w 5000g·mol^{-1})-b-poly(aspartic acid) copolymer through an acid-labile hydrazone linker (Scheme 6-4) [33]. After spontaneous self-assembly of the drug-loaded supramolecular nanocarrier, kinetic analysis clearly demonstrated the effective cleavage of the hydrazone bonds at pH<6, with concomitant release of doxorubicin. Release of doxorubicin was negligible under physiological conditions in cell culture medium (pH=7). In this case, NK911 accumulates preferentially in tumour tissue by the EPR

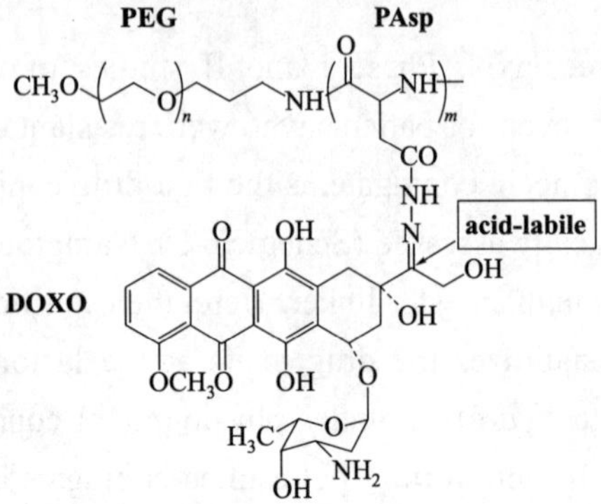

Scheme 6-4. Chemical structure of NK911.

effect, leading to a three- to four-fold improvement in targeting. And it demonstrated in vitro cytotoxicity against a human small-cell lung cancer cell line (SBC-3) in a time-dependent manner. The first candidates of antitumor drugs based on polymer micelles have entered clinical trials in Japan[34].

(4) Dendrimer-drug conjugates Dendritic polymers are synthetic, highly branched, mono-disperse macromolecules of nanometer dimensions emerged recently. Dendrimers are classified by generation, which refers to the number of repeated branching cycles that are performed during the synthesis. A dendrimer is typically symmetric around the core, and often adopts a spherical three-dimensional morphology.

Dendrimer is currently gaining much interest as dendritic nanocarriers for applications in drug delivery, due to their unique structural properties such as monodispersity, well-defined globular shape (about 20nm), high density of functional groups at periphery, multivalency and available internal cavities for drug loading. By conjugating appropriate targeting moieties, drugs and imaging agents to dendritic polymers, 'smart' drug delivery nanodevices can be developed [35].

Of the family of dendrimers, most investigated one for drug delivery is the polyamidoamine (PAMAM) dendrimer (Scheme 6-5), whose internal tertiary amines are available for acid-base interactions and hydrogen bonding with guest molecules, while the terminal amines for covalent modification of drug molecules. A PAMAM dendrimer (generation 4) N-acetyl cysteine (NAC) conjugate with a glutathione (GSH)-sensitive disulfide linker has been described for intracellular delivery of NAC in neuroinflammation treatment [36]. Drug release study indicates that the prepared PAMAM-S-S-NAC conjugate can deliver 60% of its NAC payload within 1 h at intracellular GSH concentrations at physiological pH, whereas the conjugate did not release any drug at plasma GSH levels. The conjugates showed an order of magnitude

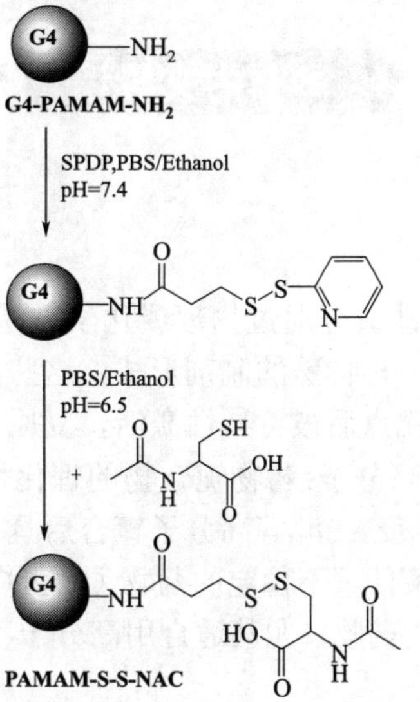

Scheme 6-5. Synthesis of dendrimer conjugates.

increase in antioxidant activity compared to free drug, in in-vitro study measured in activated microglial cells (target cells in vivo) using the reactive oxygen species (ROS) assay.

◆ **本节中文导读** ◆

高分子药物：

将高分子与药物或活性成分通过物理或化学方法轭合形成高分子-药物轭合物，也称高分子前药，是一种特殊的制剂形式。这些高分子前药在输送至靶点过程中是无活性的，在到达靶点后被特异性激活，复原成具有活性的药物成分。由于高分子的较高分子量，高分子-药物轭合物的理化性质将主要依赖于高分子本身，这也是难溶性药物与聚乙二醇等高分子轭合后具有增溶效果的重要原因。对那些非水溶性药物、生理条件下不稳定的药物（如蛋白和多肽类药物）、高毒性药物、以及难以被细胞摄取的药物，尤其适合用高分子-药物轭合物体系完成它们的体内输送。

Ringsdorf 模型中，一个理想的高分子-药物轭合物主要由高分子、生物活性组分（一种或多种药物分子）、间隔基以及靶向基团组成。高分子作为载体骨架，要具有生物相容性、无毒或低毒、无免疫原性、不会在体内积累，可以是惰性或是可降解性的；药物可直接或通过间隔基与高分子主链共价连接；间隔基以及共价键的选择要考虑轭合作用的可行性，以及之后活性药物被水解或酶解的位点和速率，通常有酯键、酰胺键和二硫键等；靶向基团用于引导高分子-药物轭合物到达人体特定的组织及细胞，靶向作用的方式有受体表达、抗体以及配体的结合等。

目前研究中涉及的高分子-药物轭合物主要包括四类：高分子-蛋白药物轭合物、高分子-抗癌药物轭合物、高分子药物轭合物胶束、树枝状大分子-药物轭合物。已有一些抗癌药物的高分子-药物轭合物陆续进入临床试验阶段，还有部分高分子生物药物轭合物已获批准上市。

6.4 Polymers for gene delivery

6.4.1 Introduction to gene delivery

Gene therapy can be defined as the treatment of human disease by the transfer of genetic material into specific cells of the patient [37]. It has gained significant attention over the past two decades as a potential method for treating many acquired and inherited life-threatening diseases, such as AIDS, cancer, genetic disorders, etc. In contrast to small drug molecules that affect the function of a target protein, the introduction of a nucleic acid drug would alter the synthesis of key proteins in selected cells by adjusting the local level of gene expression.

Here, nucleic acids usually carry a polyionic negative electric charge, and they must be delivered to the interior of the target cell in order to achieve the efficacy. Therefore, the task of delivering therapeutic nucleic acids demands a different technical approach from small molecules. Moreover, there are numerous mechanistic challenges to be overcome during the process of gene delivery, involving molecular transit from the outside medium to the cell surface, internalization, release, and distribution in the proper intracellular location [38]. In the case of DNA therapy, translocation of the DNA into the nucleus is necessary. In the case of RNA interference (RNAi), siRNA must be delivered to the RNA induced silencing complex in the cytoplasm. To achieve successful gene therapy, the development of a proper delivery vector is a key factor, which must navigate a series of obstacles, both extracellular and intracellular as mentioned above.

Nowadays, the vectors for gene delivery are usually divided into two categories: viral and nonviral (or synthetic) vectors. Though the biology of viruses provides them greater efficiency of gene delivery, nonviral vectors are preferred due to safety concerns with the viral vectors. Synthetic vectors are typically based on cationic lipids or polymers, which can complex with negatively charged nucleic acids to form particles with a diameter in the order of 100nm. Such complexes of plasmid DNA with cationic lipids and polymers are known as lipoplexes and polyplexes, respectively, which protect the nucleic acid from degradation by nuclease. In particular, polymeric gene carriers are increasingly attractive for human gene delivery because of their greater flexibility, biocompatibility and facile manufacturing [39, 40]. However, poor gene transfer efficiency limited their clinical applications. In the past decade, large amount of research has focused on designing cationic polymer system that can condense DNA and avoid both in vitro and in vivo barriers for gene delivery.

6.4.2　Polymeric vectors

Polymeric vectors are representative as cationic polymers, which comprise DNA-binding moieties such as primary, secondary, tertiary and quaternary amines, and other positively charged groups such as amidines, in the polymer backbone, in pendant groups or in grafted oligomers. The polymers themselves comprise linear, branched and dendritic structures.

Figure 6-10 represents schematically the polyplex formation by electrostatic interactions between linear polycations and DNA. When aqueous solutions of a polycation and DNA are mixed, polyplexes form spontaneously. An excess of polycation is typically used, which generates particles with a positive surface charge. Here, each particle consists of several plasmid DNA molecules and hundreds of polymer chains.

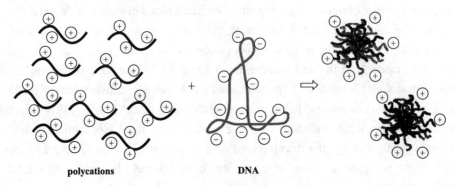

polycations　　　　　　　　DNA

Figure 6-10. Polyplex formation.

In the following section, several important classes of cationic polymers for gene delivery will be illustrated, as well as some current cellular and local delivery strategies overcoming extra- or/and intracellular barriers.

(1) Polyethylenimine (PEI)　Polyethylenimine, often considered the gold standard of gene transfection, is one of the most prominent examples of cationic polymers used in gene delivery. Since the first successful polyethylenimine-mediated oligonucleotide transfer conducted by Behr et al. in 1995 [41], a variety of PEIs and their derivates have been developed to improve the physicochemical and biological properties of polyplexes.

Polyethylenimine exists as both a branched and linear structure, as in Scheme 6-6.

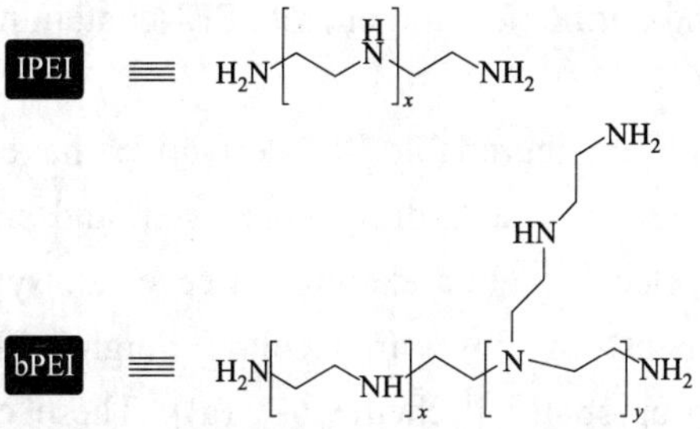

Scheme 6-6. Chemical structure of linear PEI and branched PEI.

The branching degree of polyethylenimine has been shown to affect DNA complex formation and stability. Polyplexes made from branched PEI with more primary amines usually show the higher stability [42]. Dunlap et al. showed that linear PEI is less effective in condensing DNA than the branched form with similar molecular weights [43]. However, despite the lower complexation capability of linear PEI, multiple in vivo studies have indicated linear PEI to be a particularly effective gene transfer agent due to its relative low toxicity.

The relatively high gene-transfer activity of PEI is believed to be due, at least in part, to efficient escape from the endocytic pathway through the "proton-sponge" mechanism [44]. The structure of PEI contains nitrogen at every third atom, resulting in a very high density of amines. Only $15\% \sim 20\%$ of amines are protonated at physiological pH compared to about 50% protonated nitrogens at a pH of 5, which makes PEI an extraordinarily strong proton sponge. This buffering capacity allows PEI polyplexes to avoid lysosomal trafficking and degradation once inside the cell.

Polyethylenimine with a wide range of molecular weights has been studied for transfection. Godbey et al. showed that transfection efficiency of PEI polyplexes increases with increased molecular weight ranging from 600 to 70000[45]. However, high molecular weight PEI also results in significantly higher cytotoxicity, which may be caused by aggregation and adherence of polymers on the cell surface, resulting in significant necrosis [46, 47]. The optimal molecular weight for PEI polyplex formation is typically between 5000 and 25000 [48].

To decrease cytotoxicity and enhance gene transfection efficiency, various studies [49] have derivatized PEI with either hydrophilic segments such as poly(ethylene glycol) (PEG) or hydrophobic segments such as poly(L-lactide-co-glycolide) and cholesterol, or other biocompatible compositions such as cyclodextrin. Moreover, PEI derivates have also been decorated with a variety of targeting ligands including galactose, mannose, transferrin and antibodies, to generate PEI-containing polyplexes targeted to specific cell types.

In addition, multiple biodegradable PEI derivatives have been explored with the cleavable disulfide linker or the hydrolyzable ester and imine linkages to create biodegradable gene carriers [38]. For example, Lee et al. synthesized reducible PEI derivatives by treatment of low molecular weight PEI (800) with either dithiobis(succinimidylpropionate) [Scheme 6-7 (a)]. These compounds showed less transfection efficiency than that of 25000 PEI, but exhibited significantly reduced cytotoxicity[50]. Alternatively, Pack et al. synthesized PEI derivatives with ester linkages by reacting low molecular weight branched PEI (800) with 1,3-butanediol diacrylate or 1,6-hexanediol diacrylate [Scheme 6-7 (b)]. These compounds showed significantly lower cytotoxicity and the transfection efficiency was 2~16-fold higher than 25000 PEI [51]. Kim et al. synthesized imine-linked PEI by treating low molecular weight branched PEI (1800) with glutadialdehyde [Scheme 6-7 (c)]. These structures showed reduced cytotoxicity, but the transfection efficiency was lower than that of 25000 PEI[52].

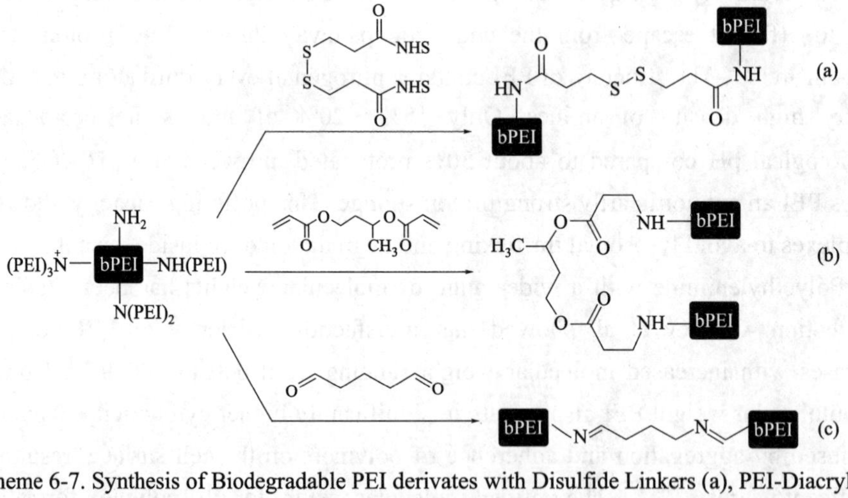

Scheme 6-7. Synthesis of Biodegradable PEI derivates with Disulfide Linkers (a), PEI-Diacrylate Derivatives by Michael Additions (b) and PEI derivates with Imine Linkers (c).

The efficacy of PEI-based delivery vectors in vivo is significantly high and animal studies demonstrate that such systems have a potential in humans. However, it should be noted that further studies involving PEI in animal models are needed so as to get a detailed toxicity profile of these vectors. Also, it is imperative that the vector reaches the specific organ causing little or no undesirable effects to other organs.

(2) Poly(L-lysine) (PLL)   Polylysine has been used for gene transfer in vitro and in vivo since it was demonstrated the exceptional capability to condense DNA by Laemmli [53]. Synthesis of PLL proceeds by conversion of an ε-amine protected L-lysine monomer to N-carboxy-(N-benzyloxycarbonyl)-L-lysine anhydride, and the anhydride undergoes ring-opening polymerization using a primary amine initiator (Scheme 6-8). Control of molecular weight can be achieved through the use of specific feed ratios of monomer to initiator. In general, only polylysine with molecular weights >3000 can effectively condense DNA to form stable complexes.

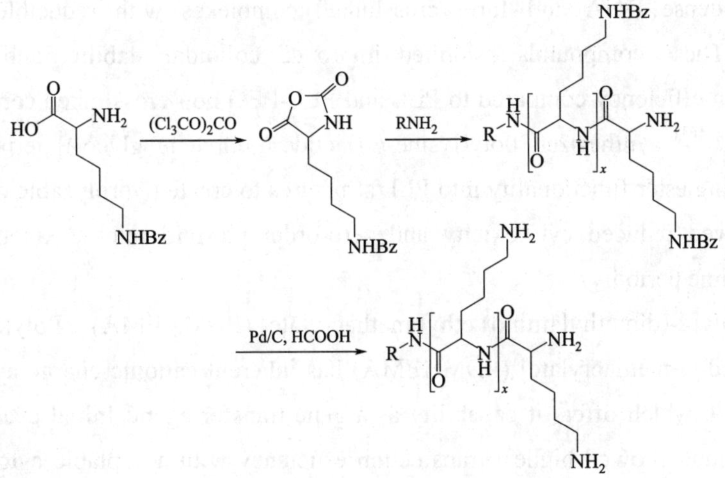

Scheme 6-8. Synthesis of Poly(L-lysine).

Despite the effective condensing ability of high molecular weight PLL, their applications in gene transfer are limited due to the relatively high cytotoxicity and the poor stability of PLL/DNA complexes, which tend to the aggregate and precipitate depending on the ionic strength of the solution. Therefore, a variety of modifications have been explored to reduce the toxicity, such as the incorporation of imidazole functionality into the poly(lysine) chain [54] as well as the use of dendritic poly(L-lysine) derivatives [55]. In addition, the attachment of PEG or dextran to PLL could prevent aggregation of PLL/DNA complexes. Kataoka et al. [56] sythesized PLL-PEG copolymers to form complexes with DNA and oligodeoxynucleotides, which showed reduced sizes regardless of the concentration of NaCl in the buffer solution and successful gene transfer.

Nevertheless, endosomal escape is a barrier for PLL/DNA complexes because all primary ε-amino groups of PLL are protonated at physiological pH, yielding a structure with no buffering capacity [57]. Endosomal release can be improved with the addition of chloroquine or membrane-active peptide[58]. An alternative method to promote endosomal lysis involves substituting PLL with histidine groups, yielding conjugate acids with a pKa=6.0, to provide PLL with buffering capacity[59].

In addition, various biodegradable polylysine conjugates have been synthesized in an effort to reduce cytotoxicity and improve release of DNA from the PLL polyplex following endocytosis. Kataoka et al. prepared thiolated PLL-*b*-PEG copolymers that could condense DNA and form crosslinked complexes with reducible disulfide linkages. These compounds exhibited improved colloidal stability and enhanced transfection efficiency compared to PLL and PLL-PEG non-crosslinked conjugates[60]. Park et al. [61] synthesized poly[lysine-g-(lactide-*b*-ethylene glycol)] terpolymer by incorporating ester functionality into PLL structures to create hydrolyzable derivatives. They showed reduced cytotoxicity and zero-order plasmid release kinetics over a six-week time period.

(3) poly[2-(dimethylamino) ethyl methacrylate] (PDMAEMA)　Poly[2-(dimethylamino) ethyl methacrylate] (PDMAEMA) has inherent cationic charge as shown in Scheme 6-9, which offers it capability as a gene transfer agent. Initial evaluations of this compound showed highest transfection efficiency with acceptable cytotoxicity at PDMAEMA/pDNA ratios of 6/1 (*w/w*) for polymer with molecular weights greater than 300000 [62]. The successful in vitro transfection efficiency of PDMAEMA polyplexes is attributed to the ability of the polymer to destabilize endosomes as well as to dissociate easily from the plasmid once delivered into the cytosol.

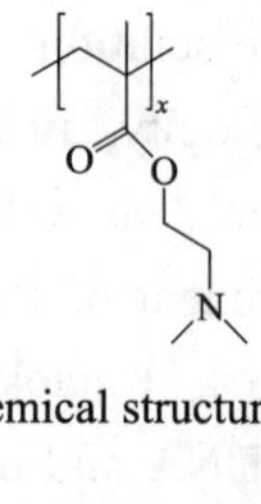

Scheme 6-9. Chemical structure of PDMAEMA.

Though in vitro investigations showed limited PDMAEMA-polyplex aggregation in the presence of albumin, significant accumulation of PDMAEMA polyplexes in the lungs was observed when they were injected intravenously into mice. It was considered to result from the formation of aggregates caused by erythrocytes[63].

(4) Polyamidoamine (PAMAM) dendrimer　PAMAM dendrimers are spheroidal and cascade polymers as shown in Figure 6-11, the size and surface charge of which can be controlled by varying the number of 'generations' in the synthesis. PAMAM dendrimers with primary amino surface groups have the inherent ability to associate, condense and efficiently transport DNA into a wide number of cell types. PAMAM dendrimers are safe and nonimmunogenic. They have become the most utilized dendrimer-based vectors for gene transfer.

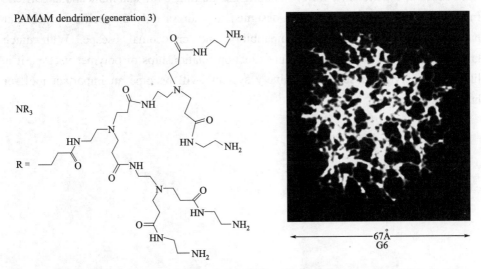

Figure 6-11. Chemical structure and molecular modeling of polyamidoamine (PAMAM) dendrimer.

Initial work using PAMAM to form a dendrimer/DNA complex (termed dendriplex) for gene transfer was conducted by Haensler and Szoka in 1993 [64]. They found that the sixth-generation dendrimer was better than higher and lower generations by about 10-fold. In general, the formation of PAMAM-based DNA complexes varies based on dendrimer/DNA charge ratio and dendrimer generation, leading to the fluctuation of transfection efficiency [65]. Due to the large number of secondary and tertiary amines on the polymer, PAMAM dendrimers are also thought to be proton sponges, which promote endosomal release of DNA in PAMAM-mediated gene delivery. Due to their relatively high gene-delivery efficiency and good biocompatibility, PAMAM dendrimers have recently been used in several in vivo gene-delivery studies [66, 67].

There are additional investigations on various alterations to the basic PAMAM dendrimer structure for improving transfection efficiency, with respect to cytotoxicity, complex formation, cell binding, endosomal release, and cell-targeting.

(5) Other polymers as gene carriers   There are many other types of polymers used in gene-delivery studies, including natrual chitosan [68], biodegradable poly(amino-ester) [69, 70] and a variety of novel polymers tailor-made for gene delivery [71]. However, polymers are generally considered unacceptable for clinical applications, since their effectiveness as gene-delivery vectors remains orders of magnitude poorer than viral vectors.   The lack of efficiency of polymer gene-delivery vectors results from a lack of functionality for overcoming the multiple extra and intracellular barriers. In most cases, the polymers were designed to address only a specific intracellular barrier, such as stability, biocompatibility and endosomal escape. With much knowledge learned about the structure-function relationships of polymer vectors, it is likely that polymer-based gene-delivery systems will become an important tool for human gene therapy.

◆ **本节中文导读** ◆

高分子基因载体：

基因治疗是一种将外源基因导入目标细胞并有效表达，从而达到治病目的的治疗方法。将治疗基因运送到目标细胞时，必须借助一种安全、稳定、转染率高的载体，但是一直以来，基因传递载体的开发却是制约基因治疗发展的瓶颈。迄今为止，用于基因输送的载体主要有病毒类载体和非病毒类载体。虽然病毒载体能获得较高的基因转染效率，但是存在安全隐患，大大限制了其临床应用。近年来被广泛研究的非病毒载体，包括阳离子脂质体和阳离子高分子材料，以其安全性、低免疫反应、靶向性及易于组装等优点被寄予厚望。

目前用于基因传递阳离子高分子主要是一些含有氨基（包括一级、二级、三级、四级胺）的正电性高分子，如：聚乙烯亚胺（PEI）、聚甲基丙烯酸二甲氨酯(PDMAEMA)、聚赖氨酸、壳聚糖等。它们可与带负电的 DNA/RNA 在水溶液中通过静电相互作用结合形成稳定的纳米复合物，有效包裹保护基因免受核酸酶降解，其正电性有助于细胞内化和内涵体逃逸，在体外细胞实验和体内动物实验中获得了一定的基因转染效果。DNA 与阳离子高分子的复合能力和基因转染率，受载体高分子材料的结构、分子量以及复合物的组分比例、形态和制备方法等因素影响很大。

如聚乙烯亚胺是目前高分子基因载体研究中应用颇为广泛的一种材料，它具有很强的质子缓冲能力，并且在多种不同细胞中均有很高的转染效率，所以被普遍当做非病毒载体的标准性物质。但聚乙烯亚胺的转染效率和细胞毒性均随分子量的增加而递增，而且其在细胞内不易降解。因此，需要开发更为安全高效的基因传递载体材料。

将治疗基因准确的输送到靶细胞的细胞核并起作用是一个相当复杂的过程，基因载体必须经历细胞外的稳定循环、靶细胞的摄取、内涵体的逃逸、细胞质内的转运、细胞核的进入和最终的基因表达等一系列障碍。尽管在过去十多年间，科学家们针对这些问题尝试了多种方法对现有阳离子高分子进行改造，或者设计合成新型刺激响应性高分子材料用作基因输送的载体，但往往只能解决部分问题。随着人们对载体材料的构效关系以及基因转染相关生物学问题的深入研究，研发安全高效的高分子基因载体具有广阔的前景。

References

[1] Kishida A and Ikada Y, Hydrogels for Biomedical and Pharmaceutical Applications, // S. Dumitriu, Editor, Polymeric Biomaterials. New York:Marcel Dekker, Inc. 2001: 113.

[2] Ratner B, Hoffman A, Schoen F, Lemons J, Biomaterials Science: An Introduction to Materials in Medicine. 2nd Ed: Academic Press, 2004.

[3] Peppas N A, Hydrogels in Medicine and Pharmacy. Boca Raton, FL: CRC Press, 1987.

[4] Hassan C M, Stewart J E, Peppas N A. Diffusional Characteristics of Freeze/Thawed Poly(Vinyl Alcohol) Hydrogels: Applications to Protein Controlled Release from Multilaminate Devices. European Journal of phormaceutics and Biopharmaceutics, 2000, 49(2): 161-165.

[5] Augst A D, Kong H J, Mooney D J. Alginate Hydrogels as Biomaterials. Macromolecular Bioscience, 2006, 6(8): 623-633.

[6] Miyata T, Uragami T, Nakamae K. Biomolecule-Sensitive Hydrogels. Advanced Drug Delivery Review Rev, 2002, 54(1): 79-98.

[7] Yuk S H, Cho S H, Lee S H. Ph/Temperature-Responsive Polymer Composed of Poly ((N, N-Dimethylamino) Ethyl Methacrylate-Co-Ethylacrylamide). Macromolecules, 1997, 30(22): 6856-6859.

[8] Loh X J and Li J. Biodegradable Thermosensitive Copolymer Hydrogels for Drug Delivery. Expert Opinion on Therapeutic Patents, 2007, 17(8): 965-977.

[9] Xia Y. Nanomaterials at Work in Biomedical Research. Nature, 2008, 7(10): 758-760.

[10] Thorley A J and Tetley T D. New Perspectives in Nanomedicine. Pharmacology & therapeutics, 2013, 140(2): 176-185.

[11] Duncan R. The Dawning Era of Polymer Therapeutics. Nature Reviews Drug Discovery, 2003, 2(5): 347-360.

[12] Nishiyama N and Kataoka K. Current State, Achievements, and Future Prospects of Polymeric Micelles as Nanocarriers for Drug and Gene Delivery. Pharmacology & therapeutics, 2006, 112(3): 630-648.

[13] Cheng Z, Al Zaki A, Hui J Z, Muzykantov V R, Tsourkas A. Multifunctional Nanoparticles: Cost Versus Benefit of Adding Targeting and Imaging Capabilities. Science, 2012, 338(6109): 903-910.

[14] Antonietti M and Göltner C. Superstructures of Functional Colloids: Chemistry on the Nanometer Scale. Angewandte Chemie International Edition in English, 1997, 36(9): 910-928.

[15] Price C. Micelle Formation by Block Copolymers in Organic Solvents. Pure and Applied Chemistry, 1983, 55(10): 1563-1572.

[16] Kataoka K, Harada A, Nagasaki Y. Block Copolymer Micelles for Drug Delivery: Design, Characterization and Biological Significance. Advanced Drug Delivery Review, 2012.

[17] Yamamoto Y, Nagasaki Y, Kato Y, Sugiyama Y, Kataoka K. Long-Circulating Poly (Ethylene Glycol) - Poly (D, L-Lactide) Block Copolymer Micelles with Modulated Surface Charge. Journal of controlled release, 2001, 77(1): 27-38.

[18] Nishiyama N, Okazaki S, Cabral H, Miyamoto M, Kato Y, Sugiyama Y, Nishio K, Matsumura Y, Kataoka K. Novel Cisplatin-Incorporated Polymeric Micelles Can Eradicate Solid Tumors in Mice. Cancer Research, 2003, 63(24): 8977-8983.

[19] Hobbs S K, Monsky W L, Yuan F, Roberts W G, Griffith L, Torchilin V P, Jain R K. Regulation of Transport Pathways in Tumor Vessels: Role of Tumor Type and Microenvironment. Proceedings of the National Academy of Sciences, 1998, 95(8): 4607–4612.

[20] Jain R K. Delivery of Molecular and Cellular Medicine to Solid Tumors. Adv Drug Deliv Rev, 2012.

[21] O'Reilly R K, Hawker C J, Wooley K L. Cross–Linked Block Copolymer Micelles: Functional Nanostructures of Great Potential and Versatility. Chemical Society Reviews, 2006, 35(11): 1068–1083.

[22] Kedar U, Phutane P, Shidhaye S, Kadam V. Advances in Polymeric Micelles for Drug Delivery and Tumor Targeting. Nanomedicine: Nanotechnology, Biology and Medicine, 2010, 6(6): 714–729.

[23] van der Meel R, Vehmeijer L J, Kok R J, Storm G, van Gaal E V. Ligand–Targeted Particulate Nanomedicines Undergoing Clinical Evaluation: Current Status. Advanced Drug Delivery Review, 2013, 65(10): 1284–1298.

[24] Cheng J, Teply B A, Sherifi I, Sung J, Luther G, Gu F X, Levy–Nissenbaum E, Radovic–Moreno A F, Langer R, Farokhzad O C. Formulation of Functionalized Plga - Peg Nanoparticles for in Vivo Targeted Drug Delivery. Biomaterials, 2007, 28(5): 869–876.

[25] Hrkach J, Von Hoff D, Ali M M, Andrianova E, Auer J, Campbell T, De Witt D, Figa M, Figueiredo M, Horhota A. Preclinical Development and Clinical Translation of a Psma–Targeted Docetaxel Nanoparticle with a Differentiated Pharmacological Profile. Science translational medicine, 2012, 4(128): 128ra39–128ra39.

[26] Cheng R, Meng F, Deng C, Klok H A, Zhong Z. Dual and Multi–Stimuli Responsive Polymeric Nanoparticles for Programmed Site–Specific Drug Delivery. Biomaterials, 2013, 34(14): 3647–3657.

[27] Vicent M J, Ringsdorf H, Duncan R. Polymer Therapeutics: Clinical Applications and Challenges for Development. Advanced Drug Delivery Review, 2009, 61(13): 1117–1120.

[28] Ringsdorf H. Structure and Properties of Pharmacologically Active Polymers. in Journal of Polymer Science: Polymer Symposia. 1975: Wiley Online Library.

[29] Vasey P A, Kaye S B, Morrison R, Twelves C, Wilson P, Duncan R, Thomson A H, Murray L S, Hilditch T E, Murray T. Phase I Clinical and Pharmacokinetic Study of Pk1 [N–(2–Hydroxypropyl) Methacrylamide Copolymer Doxorubicin]: First Member of a New Class of Chemotherapeutic Agents—Drug–Polymer Conjugates. Clinical cancer research, 1999, 5(1): 83–94.

[30] Bilim V. Technology Evaluation: Pk1, Pfizer/Cancer Research Uk. Current opinion in molecular therapeutics, 2003, 5(3): 326–330.

[31] Auzenne E, Donato N J, Li C, Leroux E, Price R E, Farquhar D, Klostergaard J. Superior Therapeutic Profile of Poly–L–Glutamic Acid–Paclitaxel Copolymer Compared with Taxol in Xenogeneic Compartmental Models of Human Ovarian Carcinoma. Clinical cancer research, 2002, 8(2): 573–581.

[32] Rowinsky E K, Rizzo J, Ochoa L, Takimoto C H, Forouzesh B, Schwartz G, Hammond L A, Patnaik A, Kwiatek J, Goetz A. A Phase I and Pharmacokinetic Study of Pegylated Camptothecin as a 1–Hour Infusion Every 3 Weeks in Patients with Advanced Solid Malignancies. Journal of clinical oncology, 2003, 21(1): 148–157.

[33] Bae Y, Fukushima S, Harada A, Kataoka K. Design of Environment - Sensitive Supramolecular Assemblies for Intracellular Drug Delivery: Polymeric Micelles That Are Responsive to Intracellular Ph Change. Angewandte Chemie International Edition, 2003, 42(38): 4640–4643.

[34] Nakanishi T, Fukushima S, Okamoto K, Suzuki M, Matsumura Y, Yokoyama M, Okano T, Sakurai Y, Kataoka K. Development of the Polymer Micelle Carrier System for Doxorubicin. Journal of controlled release, 2001, 74(1): 295–302.

[35] Patri A K, Kukowska-Latallo J F, Baker Jr J R. Targeted Drug Delivery with Dendrimers: Comparison of the Release Kinetics of Covalently Conjugated Drug and Non-Covalent Drug Inclusion Complex. Advanced Drug Delivery Review, 2005, 57(15): 2203–2214.

[36] Kurtoglu Y E, Navath R S, Wang B, Kannan S, Romero R, Kannan R M. Poly (Amidoamine) Dendrimer – Drug Conjugates with Disulfide Linkages for Intracellular Drug Delivery. Biomaterials, 2009, 30(11): 2112–2121.

[37] Mulligan R C. The Basic Science of Gene Therapy. Science, 1993, 260(5110): 926–932.

[38] Mintzer M A and Simanek E E. Nonviral Vectors for Gene Delivery. Chemical reviews, 2008, 109(2): 259–302.

[39] Ballarín-González B and Howard K A. Polyplex-Based Delivery of Rnai Therapeutics: Adverse Effects and Solutions. Advanced Drug Delivery Review, 2012.

[40] Pack D W, Hoffman A S, Pun S, Stayton P S. Design and Development of Polymers for Gene Delivery. Nature Reviews Drug Discovery, 2005, 4(7): 581–593.

[41] Boussif O, Lezoualc'h F, Zanta M A, Mergny M D, Scherman D, Demeneix B, Behr J-P. A Versatile Vector for Gene and Oligonucleotide Transfer into Cells in Culture and in Vivo: Polyethylenimine. Proceedings of the National Academy of Sciences, 1995, 92(16): 7297–7301.

[42] Reschel T, Koňák Č r, Oupický D, Seymour L W, Ulbrich K. Physical Properties and in Vitro Transfection Efficiency of Gene Delivery Vectors Based on Complexes of DNA with Synthetic Polycations. Journal of controlled release, 2002, 81(1): 201–217.

[43] Dunlap D D, Maggi A, Soria M R, Monaco L. Nanoscopic Structure of DNA Condensed for Gene Delivery. Nucleic acids research, 1997, 25(15): 3095–3101.

[44] Behr J-P. The Proton Sponge: A Trick to Enter Cells the Viruses Did Not Exploit. CHIMIA International Journal for Chemistry, 1997, 51(1–2): 1–2.

[45] Godbey W, Wu K K, Mikos A G. Size Matters: Molecular Weight Affects the Efficiency of Poly (Ethyleneimine) as a Gene Delivery Vehicle. Journal of biomedical materials research, 1999, 45(3): 268–275.

[46] Fischer D, Li Y, Ahlemeyer B, Krieglstein J, Kissel T. In Vitro Cytotoxicity Testing of Polycations: Influence of Polymer Structure on Cell Viability and Hemolysis. Biomaterials, 2003, 24(7): 1121–1131.

[47] Fischer D, Bieber T, Li Y, Elsässer H-P, Kissel T. A Novel Non-Viral Vector for DNA Delivery Based on Low Molecular Weight, Branched Polyethylenimine: Effect of Molecular Weight on Transfection Efficiency and Cytotoxicity. Pharmaceutical research, 1999, 16(8): 1273–1279.

[48] Neu M, Fischer D, Kissel T. Recent Advances in Rational Gene Transfer Vector Design Based on Poly (Ethylene Imine) and Its Derivatives. Journal of Gene Medicine, 2005, 7(8): 992–1009.

[49] Patnaik S and Gupta K C. Novel Polyethylenimine-Derived Nanoparticles for in Vivo Gene Delivery. Expert opinion on drug delivery, 2013, 10(2): 215–228.

[50] Gosselin M A, Guo W, Lee R J. Efficient Gene Transfer Using Reversibly Cross-Linked Low Molecular Weight Polyethylenimine. Bioconjugate chemistry, 2001, 12(6): 989–994.

[51] Forrest M L, Koerber J T, Pack D W. A Degradable Polyethylenimine Derivative with Low Toxicity for Highly Efficient Gene Delivery. Bioconjugate chemistry, 2003, 14(5): 934–940.

[52]   Kim Y H, Park J H, Lee M, Kim Y-H, Park T G, Kim S W. Polyethylenimine with Acid-Labile Linkages as a Biodegradable Gene Carrier. Journal of controlled release, 2005, 103(1): 209-219.

[53]   Laemmli U. Characterization of DNA Condensates Induced by Poly (Ethylene Oxide) and Polylysine. Proceedings of the National Academy of Sciences, 1975, 72(11): 4288-4292.

[54]   Putnam D, Gentry C A, Pack D W, Langer R. Polymer-Based Gene Delivery with Low Cytotoxicity by a Unique Balance of Side-Chain Termini. Proceedings of the National Academy of Sciences, 2001, 98(3): 1200-1205.

[55]   Ohsaki M, Okuda T, Wada A, Hirayama T, Niidome T, Aoyagi H. In Vitro Gene Transfection Using Dendritic Poly (L-Lysine). Bioconjugate chemistry, 2002, 13(3): 510-517.

[56]   Harada A, Togawa H, Kataoka K. Physicochemical Properties and Nuclease Resistance of Antisense-Oligodeoxynucleotides Entrapped in the Core of Polyion Complex Micelles Composed of Poly (Ethylene Glycol) - Poly (L-Lysine) Block Copolymers. European journal of pharmaceutical sciences, 2001, 13(1): 35-42.

[57]   Akinc A and Langer R. Measuring the Ph Environment of DNA Delivered Using Nonviral Vectors: Implications for Lysosomal Trafficking. Biotechnology and bioengineering, 2002, 78(5): 503-508.

[58]   Wolfert M and Seymour L. Chloroquine and Amphipathic Peptide Helices Show Synergistic Transfection in Vitro. Gene therapy, 1998, 5(3): 409.

[59]   Midoux P and Monsigny M. Efficient Gene Transfer by Histidylated Polylysine/Pdna Complexes. Bioconjugate chemistry, 1999, 10(3): 406-411.

[60]   Miyata K, Kakizawa Y, Nishiyama N, Harada A, Yamasaki Y, Koyama H, Kataoka K. Block Catiomer Polyplexes with Regulated Densities of Charge and Disulfide Cross-Linking Directed to Enhance Gene Expression. Journal of the American Chemical Society, 2004, 126(8): 2355-2361.

[61]   Park S and Healy K E. Compositional Regulation of Poly (Lysine-< I> G</I>-(Lactide-< I> B</I>-Ethylene Glycol)) - DNA Complexation and Stability. Journal of controlled release, 2004, 95(3): 639-651.

[62]   van de Wetering P, Cherng J-Y, Talsma H, Hennink W E. Relation between Transfection Efficiency and Cytotoxicity of Poly (2-(Dimethylamino) Ethyl Methacrylate)/Plasmid Complexes. Journal of controlled release, 1997, 49(1): 59-69.

[63]   Verbaan F, van Dam I, Takakura Y, Hashida M, Hennink W, Storm G, Oussoren C. Intravenous Fate of Poly (2-(Dimethylamino) Ethyl Methacrylate)-Based Polyplexes. European journal of pharmaceutical sciences, 2003, 20(4): 419-427.

[64]   Haensler J and Szoka Jr F C. Polyamidoamine Cascade Polymers Mediate Efficient Transfection of Cells in Culture. Bioconjugate chemistry, 1993, 4(5): 372-379.

[65]   Bielinska A U, Chen C, Johnson J, Baker J R. DNA Complexing with Polyamidoamine Dendrimers: Implications for Transfection. Bioconjugate chemistry, 1999, 10(5): 843-850.

[66]   Harada Y, Iwai M, Tanaka S, Okanoue T, Kashima K, Maruyama-Tabata H, Hirai H, Satoh E, Imanishi J, Mazda O. Highly Efficient Suicide Gene Expression in Hepatocellular Carcinoma Cells by Epstein-Barr Virus-Based Plasmid Vectors Combined with Polyamidoamine Dendrimer. Cancer gene therapy, 2000, 7(1): 27-36.

[67]   Maruyama-Tabata H, Harada Y, Matsumura T, Satoh E, Cui F, Iwai M, Kita M, Hibi S, Imanishi J, Sawada T. Effective Suicide Gene Therapy in Vivo by Ebv-Based Plasmid Vector Coupled with Polyamidoamine Dendrimer. Gene therapy, 2000, 7(1): 53-60.

[68] Mao S, Sun W, Kissel T. Chitosan-Based Formulations for Delivery of DNA and Sirna. Advanced Drug Delivery Review, 2010, 62(1): 12-27.

[69] Lynn D M, Anderson D G, Putnam D, Langer R. Accelerated Discovery of Synthetic Transfection Vectors: Parallel Synthesis and Screening of a Degradable Polymer Library. Journal of the American Chemical Society, 2001, 123(33): 8155-8156.

[70] Zugates G T, Anderson D G, Little S R, Lawhorn I E, Langer R. Synthesis of Poly (B-Amino Ester) S with Thiol-Reactive Side Chains for DNA Delivery. Journal of the American Chemical Society, 2006, 128(39): 12726-12734.

[71] Zhou J, Liu J, Cheng C J, Patel T R, Weller C E, Piepmeier J M, Jiang Z, Saltzman W M. Biodegradable Poly (Amine-Co-Ester) Terpolymers for Targeted Gene Delivery. Nature materials, 2011, 11(1): 82-90.